TREATING FEVER Without Fear

by
Robyn Barraclough and Molly Knight

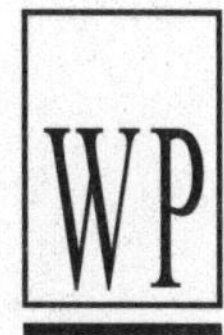

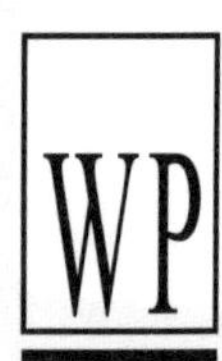

Published by Wilkinson Publishing Pty Ltd
ACN 006 042 173
PO Box 24135, Melbourne, VIC 3000, Australia
Ph: +61 3 9654 5446
enquiries@wilkinsonpublishing.com.au
www.wilkinsonpublishing.com.au

Disclaimer

The information we provide in this book is not meant to replace your doctor's care or treatment protocol. It is not intended to diagnose, treat, cure or prevent any health problem or condition. It is sensible and advisable that you consult with your health care professional before you decide to use any of the remedies or techniques contained within these pages. Never delay getting medical advice because of something you have read in this book.

ISBN: 9781921667862

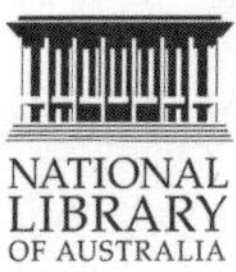

A catalogue record for this book is available from the National Library of Australia

Cover and internal design by Alicia Freile, Tango Media

Printed and bound in Australia by Ligare.

Follow Wilkinson Publishing on social media.

 WilkinsonPublishing

 wilkinsonpublishinghouse

 WPBooks

Dedicated to every mother, grandmother, parent or carer who feels that pang of anxiety, helplessness and fear when their child is ill or in pain, and they don't know what to do.

Table of Contents

Introduction

First Steps to Taking Control of Your Family's Health

Thank you for purchasing our book. We have written this book to pass on the information that we believe will be helpful to you, as a front-line home healer. We know you will find the information useful and practical to use.

The purpose of writing this book is to give you the immediate steps to take when faced with an acute health issue, and in doing so you can change the trajectory of how the body responds to illness. These steps will not suppress or mask symptoms but instead activate the natural healing ability of the immune system. By giving our suggested remedies at the onset of an illness, you begin the healing process and potentially reduce the severity and longevity of any illness.

This book does not replace responsible medical intervention. However, by taking these steps you will learn several things:

1. How you can support your family when they become sick, and help them be healthier, naturally.
2. How to recognise the early signs of illness and what to do about it.
3. How to look for the cause of the fever and start to recognise the different ways that the body is telling you what is wrong, and what it needs.
4. By noticing these simple signs, you can support your child more effectively should they need medical attention, by clearly describing their symptoms to your doctor, naturopath or appropriate health care practitioner.

When you are empowered with a solid knowledge of Herbs, Homeopathy, Tissue salts, Essential Oils, Vitamins and Minerals, you can be a proactive healer in your home. You will hold the tools to promote vitality and health.

CHAPTER 1

A Parent's Guide to Natural Remedies for Children's Health

We are both very passionate about sharing our years of experience and knowledge and passing information on to people so that they may look after their health and that of their children in a natural and healthy manner.

As parents, we always want the best for our children. We strive to create a happy and healthy family and enjoy all opportunities doing all the things we love to do. We all want good health, and we want our kids to be fit, healthy and happy. In an ideal world, we would love to be bullet-proof and not succumb to any illness at all! This, sad but true, is a fantasy! It's just not possible, as you will always be getting a 'bug' or two each year. This is actually an excellent thing!

Each time your child gets an infection, a cough, a cold or a tummy bug, they build up their immune response and learn how to fight whatever comes their way. It takes time and many experiences with different pathogens for the body to build adequate resistance to illness. For example, if your child is bullied in the playground, do you want them to cower and collapse in the corner, or do you want them to be able to stand up for themselves, in a strong, assertive manner? This ability to stand strong doesn't happen overnight. You learn how to respond to a bully, by interactions, and discover when to stand your ground and when to walk away. Similarly, the body learns how to fight infections, bugs, viruses, or unwanted invaders by coming into contact with them and then activating the immune system to fight and build a remembered response, so that the next time it comes in contact with that bug or something similar it knows what to do to fight it. This response from their body indicates that they have a healthy immune system that is able to respond to an invader.

You want your child's body and their immune system maintained in a robust and healthy state, dealing with any intruders quickly and easily. This allows their body to build a natural immunity to the current bugs doing the rounds, with their body bouncing back to good health with minimal adverse effect, and without becoming overly debilitated.

To keep their immune response active, you need to look at your family's lifestyle and diet, which are the first steps to developing a healthy, fully responsive and robust immune system for your child. You will need to be proactive and practice some preventative measures to allow everyone's body to deal with any bugs that come lurking your family's way. The good news is that there is so much you can do by utilising natural remedies to keep your family healthy and full of vitality.

The human body is such a miracle, continually healing and rebalancing itself. When you bump yourself and get a bruise, you don't physically do anything, yet your body is busy healing the area. If you cut yourself or get a graze on your skin, without thinking about it, your body will heal the area with a scab, and in a few days, you won't even notice the damage. When a bone is broken, the only thing that can be done by doctors is to realign the bone and set it in plaster so it doesn't move. There is no actual intervention by man to heal the bone. The body does all the healing. We just need to give it the fuel that it requires to do all this work. Like we said, this body of ours is a miracle!

These days, we live in such a fast-paced, chemically laden world that our poor old body is constantly working hard just to stay upright and moving, let alone having the extra burden of working to banish any infectious bugs. Our body needs our help!

Your immune system is constantly on alert. Just like an army, ever ready for what may come its way. Your job is to give your body all the required support that your immune system needs to be fully active and strong. You want an immune system full of healthy active soldiers, like SAS or Seals, and not the foot soldiers wearily walking the perimeter!

Our hope is that this book will help you on your journey to health and that you will adopt some of the suggestions we have given. With over 60 years of clinical practice between us, and as parents ourselves, we know that these remedies and the strategies suggested will work for you. All tried and true. All you have to do is implement them.

CHAPTER 2

What is Fever

Hippocrates, in the 5th century BC, was probably one of the first to understand the importance of fever as part of the immune response. He is quoted as having said 'Give me a fever and I will cure all disease'. What does that mean, and how can fever cure a disease?

Let's have a look at what fever is.

Pretty simple really! Fever is the body heating up.

In general, fever is defined as an elevated body temperature above your normal temperature range due to an altered Hypothalamic set point.

What does this mean?

We certainly aren't taught this, and we rarely ever think about how our internal body continually functions. It is fascinating to realise that your body temperature is never static and changes many times in the day! Technology, like Smart Watches and Rings, allows us to track these normal body variations which previously had to be measured by a thermometer throughout the day.

Your body has a normal temperature range that is unique to you. The hypothalamus is a gland in your brain that regulates a lot of metabolic processes. When you get a fever, your body raises its temperature. The hypothalamus sets a peak temperature that it knows has the best opportunity to fight the invading pathogens. At the same time, your body triggers the immune system to activate T-killer cells and macrophages to eliminate the offending pathogens. When the immune system has effectively dealt with the invading pathogens, the body will naturally regulate back to normal temperature.

The normal body temperature is around 37°C. It can vary from person to person and can vary during the day and night.

You can feel when your child is a bit warmer than usual, or even see it in their face, with rosy cheeks that feel warm to touch. You know they have a fever, and it is usually the first indicator that they are fighting a bug of some kind, or something internally or emotionally is out of balance.

It is important to know that fever is a vital healing defence of the body.

A rise in temperature is merely a symptom that shows us the degree of severity of what is happening on the inside of the body.

Unlike giving paracetamol with the intention to bring down or stop a fever, when we suggest remedies, our main focus is to facilitate the body's own ability to deal with any infection or imbalance that may cause the core body temperature to rise.

The advantage of using our suggested protocol of remedies is that no matter the cause of the rise in temperature, the remedies support the body's ability to heal and rebalance.

CHAPTER 3

Where Did the Fear of Fever Come From?

Today, in our western culture, we have been conditioned to believe that a fever is a bad thing, that it's scary and has to be suppressed or gotten rid of as soon as possible. Believing the very false notion that if we get the fever down and back to normal, the illness is on the way out.

This is so far from the truth that it is scary! The exact opposite is really the truth. When you stop a fever, you stop the body from healing. When the body has developed a naturally fevered state, the body then goes to work, via secreting antiviral and antibacterial chemicals called Interferons. In this action, the body increases its white blood cells, both in their number and their ability to move around and do the job they are designed for.

So where did this fear of fever come from?

Interestingly, as early as the 2nd century AD physicians were advocating fever as part of the body's way to help cure diseases. The great Ancient Greek Physician Hippocrates claimed, "Those that cannot be cured by [medicine or] surgery can be cured by heat; and those that cannot be cured by heat are considered incurable".

So why did the perspective change?

Before modern medicine evolved, one possibility is that fever was often associated with people getting really sick. Watching someone with a fever and not knowing what to do can be scary. In past centuries, less was known about the body and how it worked. Common people, with very few resources to call for any form of medical help, would have seen family members and friends who became ill, get a high fever, never recover and die. The fever was thought to have caused the death.

Throughout most of history, fever has been viewed with fear, because people did not understand its role in the body. Fever was seen to be the foe rather than the underlying infection that was causing the fever. People didn't die of the fever, but of the infection that was going on inside the body. But what they could see and feel was the fever, so the fear developed from a lack of knowledge.

Now we have the research that supports the fact that it is not the fever itself that causes the illness or death, it is what is hidden from view, the pathogens that cause the illness.

Nowadays, the greatest fear medically regarding infantile fevers amongst doctors are febrile seizures where death or brain damage were the most serious complications if a fever went over 40 Degrees Celsius. Whilst the chance of this is low and associated with the cause of the fever rather than the fever itself, doctors started prescribing medications to bring down all fevers with drugs like paracetamol and ibuprofen, even for low fevers, although the risks for febrile seizures were actually for high fevers. However, just because you have a high fever does not mean that you are at high risk of febrile seizures.

> "Febrile seizures may be alarming and upsetting to witness but they are not harmful to your child. Even long

seizures lasting an hour or more almost never cause harm. Febrile seizures do not cause brain damage there is no increased risk of epilepsy in children that have had febrile seizures. Most children with fever suffer only minor discomfort however 1 child in 30 will have a febrile seizure as a result of fever. Febrile seizures most commonly happen between the ages of 6 months and 6 years. Usually children who have a febrile seizure will only ever have just one. Treating a Childs fever with paracetamol or ibuprofen will not prevent a febrile seizure."

The Royal Childrens Hospital Melbourne. Information Febrile Seizures.
https:/www.rch.aug.au/kidsinfo/fact_sheets/ febrile_convulsions/

Suppress Fever, or Let It Ride? That Is The Question...

There are two camps about how to treat fever. 'Suppress' or 'Let It Ride'.

Suppress Fever Camp

The 'suppression' camp advocates getting a fever down and keeping it down. The problem with this, is that the body doesn't ever reach and hold the correct temperature to eliminate the pathogens of an infection.

Let It Ride Camp

The 'Let it ride' camp advocates letting the fever ride it's course, as 'fever is a protective mechanism with benefits ranging from enhancing immune-cell function to promoting antimicrobial activity.'

Be Proactive with Fever Camp

There is actually another step to the "let it ride" camp, which is *Be Proactive with Fever*. What we mean by this is that by taking action using the natural remedies we outline in this book, you can let a fever ride, AND 'Be Proactive', treating the cause of the inflammation, infection or whatever is causing the fever, therefore speeding up the passage of the fever.

This reduces the risk of complications and starts the healing of the disease process that caused the fever in the first place.

CHAPTER 4

Types of Fever

A fever is just getting hot, right? You might think that but no. There are actually six main types of fevers. In our experience, when we treat fever in the way outlined in this book, we rarely see the fever continue beyond the first 24 hours, so we usually don't get to see fevers going into the full range of these fever patterns.

You or your family may not be in situations to experience all these types of fever or experience the types of diseases that they occur in, but if you see these fever patterns, you will know they are just that, patterns, which provide information. By having this information and knowledge, if you need to see a health professional, you will be more informed, and able to communicate more effectively what is happening with your child which makes it easier for your practitioner to diagnose what's wrong and consequently may be able to help you more effectively.

TYPE 1: CONTINUOUS FEVER or SUSTAINED FEVER

Continuous fever is the type of fever that most people commonly think of when we talk about fever. This fever is prolonged, and the temperature doesn't change much, if at all over the course of the day. Over the course of 24 hours, the temperature remains elevated above normal and doesn't fluctuate more than 1 degree Celsius.

Diseases with this fever type:

Pneumonia, urinary tract infections and typhoid have this type of fever. Typhoid may show up as a step ladder pattern, in a stepwise pattern which means that the fever will increase then plateau, then increase than plateau. This is rarely seen in western countries but if you are travelling, you may see it in third world countries.

ROBYN'S CASE STUDY

My daughter, aged 5 years old, would often wake up screaming in the middle of the night from nightmares, talking without being fully conscious, with a high fever and a flushed face. The bed sheets would be strewn asunder, she would often be down at the foot of the bed instead of the top, sitting bolt-upright with a 39˚C or higher temperature. On initial observation my daughter presented as a typical Belladonna case, however due to the restlessness and the nightmares, I gave her Aconite and within minutes she settled and fell asleep. By morning she was no longer feverish and was settled, calm and her normal self.

TYPE 2: INTERMITTENT FEVER

Intermittent fever starts out high but falls to normal (37.2^{0} C or below each day). In this type of fever, you may feel like you are getting better then the fever returns.

Diseases with this fever type:

Tuberculosis, Parasite infection, Lymphoma, Septicaemia

Malaria - if you travel to the tropics or subtropics in areas where malaria is common, and get bitten by mosquitoes, the first signs of infection may be an intermittent fever.

MOLLY'S CASE STUDY

A boy of 11 presented with an enlarged lymph node, and had suffered for several weeks with a fever that would come and go. He had many medical tests, but they could not find a reason for these ongoing symptoms.

When I first saw him, he was pleasant but wary, a bit over all the tests he had endured. He had a very pale face and a noticeable enlarged lymph gland on the back of his neck. His mother was feeling fearful and felt sure the enlarged lymph node would lead to something sinister.

I had previously dealt with a child who had experienced fevers coming and going, again no medical diagnosis had been found. This child was younger and had a very rounded tummy, with a few slightly enlarged lymph nodes. The first step I took was to treat her for worms, which resolved with a positive outcome.

Drawing on this experience, and considering the medical tests hadn't shown anything, I felt treating this boy for parasites might help and certainly would do no harm.

He was prescribed a Herbal Remedy, some Tissue Salts and Homeopathic remedies. Within 3 weeks the enlarged neck gland had returned to normal size, and the fevers had ceased.

At the follow-up consultation, he had a lot more colour in his face, he was smiling and obviously felt better in himself. There was no enlarged lymph gland visible or palpable, and his temperature was normal.

TYPE 3: REMITTENT FEVERS

In Remittent Fever, the body temperature fluctuates, but even when it falls, it never falls all the way back to normal body temperature.

Diseases with this fever type:

Infectious diseases such as infective endocarditis, rickets, brucellosis and many other infections, have this type of fever.

ROBYN'S CASE STUDY

Fever before getting on an aeroplane.

On the way to the airport in London, an hour-long trip in a cab, my daughter started feeling warm and complaining of an earache. A few days earlier she had had a slight fever which had dropped and I thought nothing more of it. As we drove on, she started getting more upset and Chamomile made no difference. I started to wonder if we would need to cancel our return flight to Australia to another day, even though we were scheduled to fly in a few hours. I remembered that Medorhinum is a good remedy when travelling, for balancing pressure in the ears. I gave her a dose of Medorrhinum 200C. Her fever settled and she was calm for the whole trip, including multiple take offs and landings, all the way to Sydney. It was only on the bus trip home to Canberra that she started to whimper again. I repeated Medorrhinum 200C and although she was still a bit unsettled, once she got home to her own bed and had a good sleep, she had no further issues.

TYPE 4: HECTIC FEVER

In Hectic Fever, there are wide swings in temperature. Intermittent or remittent fever types are considered hectic if there is a temperature difference of more than

1.4 degrees Celsius between the lowest and highest temperatures.

Diseases with this fever type:

Abscesses and pyogenic infections can cause this kind of fever. Pyogenic infections are pus-producing infections that occur when a wound becomes infected or in diseases like pyelonephritis.

ROBYN'S CASE STUDY

I treated a client that had a really nasty tooth infection from an abscess under a tooth. I gave her Aconite and Silica, which helped to manage the fever and pain until she could get to her dentist and have the offending damaged tooth removed and the underlying infection resolved.

TYPE 5: RELAPSING FEVER

This is a type of intermittent fever. The fever may resolve but then recur again after days or weeks of normal temperatures.

Diseases with this fever type:

It is most common with animal bites or diseases like malaria.

ROBYN'S CASE STUDY

This is another one of my children, (I have had a great deal of experience with childhood fevers, I have 5 beautiful children!) With my first daughter, I had not yet become a practitioner although I did see a herbalist and a homeopath for health issues. Every month my daughter would get a green slimy runny nose, blocked ears with a mild fever occurring. I would get that dreaded call from daycare and I would have to leave work to keep her at home. My homeopath tried many different remedies for her, and nothing really made a lasting difference, until she was given the Tissue Salt Calc Sulph. We had tried the homeopathic Calc Sulph with some success but not until the actual Tissue Salt was given, did we experience complete resolution.

Once I saw the dramatic change with this Tissue Salt, I went on to do further study of the Institute of Biochemic Medicine (Asia-Pacific) and I started to use more of the Tissue Salts with my other children with outstanding results and become a teacher as I understood the benefits of these simple and often overlooked remedies.

As a teen, my daughter started to suffer with dizziness and mild fever. Initially I gave her Ferr Phos, but when I realised these symptoms were recurring and based on my previous experience with her, I gave her Calc Sulph Tissue Salt, and she recovered and there were no further recurrences.

TYPE 6: FEBRILE SEIZURES

Some children have febrile seizures or febrile convulsions. This is very frightening for the parents. These seizures happen in 2-4% of children under 5 years old.

2.4 - 5% of children who have febrile seizures go on to develop epilepsy. Febrile seizures are most likely to occur when a child has a fever above 38 degrees Celsius, (100.4 degrees Fahrenheit), but occasionally febrile seizures may occur before a fever even begins.

If your child has febrile seizures or convulsions along with fever, it is important to consult a health professional.

Recently there have been studies about the relationship of fever and febrile convulsions.

The evidence is pointing towards a connection to a family history of and genetic predisposition to febrile seizures being the major factor in a child having recurring febrile convulsions, whereas if there is no family history of febrile seizures, the likelihood of future febrile convulsions is rare.

Additionally, there is abundant evidence that using fever reducing medications has no effect on preventing further febrile seizures.

Numerous studies show that if a child has a febrile seizure when their fever is greater than 40°C it is highly unlikely they will have another febrile seizure. Whereas, a child who has a seizure at a low temperature has a lower tolerance of fever and may be susceptible to recurrent seizures, if they have a genetic predisposition.

Consequently, contrary to popular opinion, a high temperature at the start of a febrile convulsion is a useful indicator that the febrile convulsion is unlikely to happen again.

CHAPTER 5

Symptoms of Fever

The key symptom of fever is a temperature over 38° Celsius.

Depending on the cause of the fever, these are some of the symptoms that your child may have with the fever:

- Headaches often accompany fever - these may be experienced as painful or a throbbing sensation
- Shivering and feeling cold when no one else feels cold
- Muscle aches and pains which may be sharp or dull or a constant ache
- Sweating is the body's natural response to help cool the extremities of the body once the appropriate temperature to fight an infection has been reached
- Restlessness which may be due to uncomfortable body sensations, emotional agitation or anxiety
- Weakness or fatigue, as the body fights the pathogen, toxins are released from the cells. If these aren't eliminated quickly, the dying pathogens and dead cells create debris in the blood system whilst the body tries to muster the required nutrients and energy to eliminate them.
- Rashes anywhere on the body may appear. A variety of different red rashes or bumps or specific blisters may appear during or after the fever in the case of many childhood diseases like chicken pox, measles etc.
- Increased sensitivity to pain, because the body is in a state of high alert, any experience can be more acute.

- Signs of Dehydration may be noticed as the body has stoked the internal fires, created heat, and used a lot of energy. If you don't drink enough water to counteract the effect of the fever then dehydration can occur.
- Low appetite and digestion are most effective when we are resting, but in fever, most of the body's energy is taken up with fighting the infection. The body's nervous system is in Fight Mode, which turns off digestion. Therefore, appetite is reduced as the energy is taken away from the digestive tract for the other more important tasks of fighting pathogens or invaders.
- Lack of energy and feeling sleepy, although it may not look like it from the outside, when there is a fever, your body is using an enormous amount of internal and cellular energy to fight off any infection and process the toxins and byproducts of fever. It's hard work, so of course your body wants to rest, and will in a sense demand rest, so feeling tired and sleepy is normal.
- Difficulty in concentrating even when reading a book your child loves, as the energy is sent elsewhere for healing and other functions that a back seat.

If a baby has a fever, these symptoms may be prominent

- They feel hot to touch
- Flushed cheeks
- Sweaty
- With high fever, there may be irritability, delirium, confusion or in very rare cases, seizures.

CHAPTER 6

Normal Body Temperature

Normal body temperature is the result of a balance of heat production and heat loss. The hypothalamus, a gland in the brain, helps regulate the temperature and acts as the body's thermostat, monitoring this balance. Even in healthy conditions, the body temperature naturally fluctuates, being lower in the morning and higher in the late afternoon and evening.

- Normal body temperature of a child - to 37.4°C/ 97°C - 99.4°C
- Normal body temperature of an adult – 37°C / 98.6°C
- An oral body temperature above 38°C is considered a fever. And if it goes above 40°C it is serious. A fever will generally self-resolve in a few days.

There are several factors, apart from having an infectious bug, that can cause the temperature to be raised one or two degrees:

- consuming hot food
- participating in recent exercise
- stress or excitement
- emotional distress
- wearing clothes that are not temperature appropriate
- a hot day can cause the body temperature to rise
- overheated rooms

Children often have their lowest temperature of the day early in the morning, and the highest temperature in the early evening and during the wee hours after midnight. This is the same for adults, as it is the normal rhythm of the body. So, without any infections going on in the body, a child will naturally feel a little warmer in the early evening and during the night.

It is a good idea to know where your healthy child's temperature sits. Every day at the same time for about a week, when your child is in good health, take your child's temperature and record it. You will probably find that each of your children is a bit different in their base temperature range.

Celsius - Fahrenheit conversion:

Celsius	Fahrenheit
35.6	96
36.1	97
36.7	98
37.2	99
37.8	100
38.3	101
38.9	102
39.4	103
40.0	104
40.6	105

Temperature can be taken under the arm, orally in the mouth or by the new non-contact thermometers. The temperature will vary slightly from one area to the next, so make sure you use the same area and thermometer when taking a temperature. Don't do it under the arm in the morning and then orally in the afternoon. An oral temperature is generally thought to be the most accurate and is often a bit higher than one taken under the arm.

CHAPTER 7

What Causes Fever?

Generally a fever is the body's response to a viral, bacteria or fungal infection, that has occurred because of a lowered body resistance. This can happen for many reasons. Too much sugar in the diet, a child being overactive and not getting enough rest, or a child might be a really fussy eater and is not getting adequate nutrients into their body.

It may even be that your child has been fighting off a bug, with little or no obvious signs, and the body then heats up to remove the toxic materials left over. No matter the reason for the lowered resistance, a fever is an indication that the body is working as it needs to, to restore itself back to health.

WHAT CAUSES AN INCREASE IN TEMPERATURE?

If a child feels hot after consuming hot food, participating in recent exercise, wearing clothes that are not suited to the temperature of the day, if it's a really hot day, they are in an overheated room, or emotionally distressed, disturbed or overexcited, your child may feel hot, but as these situations are each addressed your child will cool down, and you will know they are not brewing any infectious bug.

If your child feels hot and is obviously not well, they most likely are fighting a bug, however, a child can be fighting off a bug and have a fever yet still be full of energy and running around. Everyone is different.

So many of our infectious diseases start off with exactly the same symptoms. For example, if your child has a fever, a runny nose, a bit of a cough, or maybe a sore throat, you might be thinking your child is coming down with a cold. However, it could also be any one of the following illnesses:

- Measles
- Rubella
- Influenza
- Seasonal allergies
- Food allergies
- Erythema Infectiosum (slapped cheek)
- Polio
- Hand, Foot & Mouth disease
- Chickenpox
- Glandular fever
- Cytomegalovirus
- RSV

Other causes of fever:

- Infections in surgical wounds, open wounds or dental abscesses under a tooth
- Teething in babies can cause a fever
- Viral or bacterial infections are the most common cause of fever. This includes colds, flu, gastroenteritis or infection in the ears, skin, throat or bladder.
- Heat stroke or extreme sunburn
- Hormonal disorders (more common in older teenage children)
- Drugs or drug side effects, and drug withdrawal
- Inflammatory diseases such as Rheumatoid arthritis, Lupus, Irritable Bowel Syndrome (IBS)
- Cancerous growth

A fever will occur when the body considers something to be a foreign invader. This may be viruses, bacteria, fungi, heavy metals, drugs or toxins and the body considers these invaders to be pyrogens (pathogenic fever-producing substances). The hypothalamus receives a signal that these fever-producing substances are present and so raises the body temperature set point in order to kill off the pathogens. The body starts shivering to produce more heat and restricts heat loss by closing the pores until the body reaches its set point, then opens the pores, allowing the resulting sweat to cool the body.

Obviously, with some of these illnesses, other symptoms will develop soon after the fever kicks in. But you get the idea. As soon as you see any symptoms develop, you can start to address them with Herbs, Tissue Salts, Homeopathic Remedies, good healing foods and lots of rest. When you support the body's own immune response and give it the extra boost it needs to mount a large-scale defence, you can often avoid a deep infection.

CHAPTER 8

Is Fever a Friend or Foe?

Fever, like pain, is most definitely your friend! A very good friend. In fact, for your child, it is their BFF! Fever is the indicator that the immune system is working properly; it has detected an intruder and has activated all the healing mechanisms that are required so the body can heal itself.

Acute symptoms are very important for our body. Inflammation heats the body up to kill off the pathogen. It is a part of our healing response, and a fever that runs its natural course, is one of our greatest allies, stimulating the healing responses of our body.

Today, in our Western culture, we have been conditioned to believe that a fever is a bad thing, that it's scary and has to be suppressed or gotten rid of as soon as possible. Believing the very false notion that if we get the fever down and back to normal, the illness is on the way out.

This is so far from the truth that it is scary! The exact opposite is really the truth. When you stop a fever, you stop the body from healing. When the body has developed a naturally fevered state, the body then goes to work, via secreting antiviral and antibacterial chemicals called Interferons. In this action, the body increases its white blood cells, both in their number and their ability to move around.

This is how your body will heal. The immune system is doing its job, heating the body up to kill the bugs. Most pathogens or bugs (colloquial terms for viruses, bacteria etc) need a specific range of temperature for survival and multiplication. When the body heats up it renders the environment too hot for these bugs to survive in, but the temperature is perfect for the army of your own immune killer cells that are released to go forth and kill the invaders. And so, the little nasties die off. A perfect system!

So, when you take medications to lower the body temperature, the innate intelligence of your body assumes you no longer need these antiviral or antibacterial chemicals and eventually stops releasing them. This lengthens the time it takes to heal, and worse than that, the act of taking these suppressive medications can send the bacteria or virus deeper into the body, where it will simply sit and wait for its next attack.

Paracetamol, or similar over-the-counter medications, will certainly bring down a fever. But at a cost. The most damaging action that occurs is the suppression of the body's natural healing response. A lot of the infections of childhood actually need the fever to burn off the infection, so that the body can resolve its ability to function properly. Fever is only an issue if it is at a high level for a prolonged period of time. Consequently, we want to support the body to have what it needs for the fever to pass quickly.

Remember, there will always be bugs, or pathogens floating around. This is how your child's immune system learns and develops, which takes until around puberty to fully mature. So, you want your child in contact with the bugs, playing in the dirt and getting the cold. What you don't want is your child getting really sick and debilitated. This is where our protocols for dealing with fever and illness will serve you well.

Interestingly, have you noticed how a child who has been protected from contact with bugs by having little contact outside the family can maintain good health? When they go to childcare, they seem to contract every bug around as their body races to build up their immunity. If each time they get sick the illness is suppressed, the parent ends up with a child on the merry-go-round of sickness. However, if you use the tips in this book to build up the immune system, you will see the episodes reduce in frequency and duration when they are exposed to illness.

Robyn, having 5 children herself, has seen many instances where the children have gone to bed either with a fever, or waking at night with a fever, the appropriate remedies have been given, and they are better by morning. These natural remedies are not suppressing the fever, but supporting the body with what it needs so the fever can do its job and pass quickly.

CASE STUDY

One of Robyn's children woke up with an extreme earache one night.

I was woken around midnight by my 10-year-old daughter. She was holding her ear and crying in pain. "'I need the oil," she told me in between the pain.

Immediately I knew she had a really bad earache again. She used to get severe earaches a lot when she was younger. I touched her forehead, she was hot. Due to the intensity of her pain and her fever, I gave the appropriate homeopathic remedy every 10 minutes. I settled her into a comfortable position and put mullein oil in her ear to help her body with the infection. I could feel that her body was settling incrementally with each dose of the remedies.

Her father however had woken up and was getting anxious. I was confident in what I was doing and that it was working, but he started getting fearful so wanted to give her paracetamol. I don't normally have paracetamol like Panadol in the house, and have always treated my kids naturally, however, her dad had purchased some previously because he always felt so fearful when they were sick. I could see that if he gave her a dose, it would allay his fears, and I could get on with treating her, and would have the opportunity to see how the medication affected the process. Kaitlin was at an age where she could tell me she wanted to try it. So, we did. He found the paracetamol and gave her a dose. For the next 30 minutes, I noticed a plateau in the healing process.

Previously, each time I gave a remedy, I noticed the intensity of the symptoms diminishing. After the paracetamol, the process slowed from what had become a really dynamic process using the remedies up till that point. I continued using the remedies, and shortly after she settled, I slept with her that night, with one hand on her ear, comforting her. Once the paracetamol wore off, her fever rose again, and she asked for more drops in her ear. I repeated the Homeopathic remedies. The next morning she woke up with the pain gone. She rested the following day, but neither the fever nor the earache recurred.

Today I asked her about that episode and what helped. She said that she asked for the oil because it always helped, but she felt the paracetamol didn't help her pain.

It is interesting that over the last winter here down under, doctors were in the media, publicly saying not to give children anything to bring down a fever. Finally, they are catching up to what we (yes natural healers!) have been saying for decades. Let the fever follow its own course.

The other important factor to remember is to assess how sick your child physically looks (e.g., drowsy, lethargic, not playful, not smiling). This is in fact more important than how high the fever is or the number showing on your thermometer.

Remember, fever is the messenger, not the enemy. You know what they say, don't kill the messenger as these symptoms are our internal messengers!

CHAPTER 9

Treating a Fever

There are some simple steps you can take to keep your child comfortable while their body heats up and fights off a bug. It is important that you look at the overall picture of your child.

If they have a fever around 38°C but are eating and drinking well and are happy to play, you can just keep watching them to see how they go.

Suppose, however, they are off their food, and don't want to drink, and are a bit whingy and obviously unwell. In that case, if the fever has been going for a couple of days, and you have done everything you can and given them all the natural support remedies, then it's time to see your doctor.

This is a judgement call by you, the parent, and you know your child better than any health professional ever will, so never feel bad to take a child to a doctor or emergency department of a hospital, even if their temperature starts to drop within a short space of time after seeking medical help. Better to be cautious when you know you have done all you can. Mostly a fever will dissipate after a few days or sooner with remedies, but it can be very worrying for the parents. We know!

If your child is under 3 months of age, always see your doctor if they have any high fevers at all. Don't delay!

Simple steps to treat fever

- Keep your child relaxed
- Don't cover them with blankets
- Use layers of clothes that they can take off or put on as they feel warmer or cool down
- Give cool drinks, but not cold drinks, and certainly not soda pop or commercial fruit juices
- Give water to drink

Previous protocols included:

- a gentle fan in the room to keep the air circulating
- Sponging down with a cool cloth or a cool bath

Current protocols don't recommend this, rather let the body regulate naturally.

Children instinctively know what they need. Just like Robyn's story of her daughter coming in and asking for the oil for her ear. She knew that would make her feel better. Your job as a parent is to play detective and work out what your child needs based on your knowledge and what your child is asking for.

If a child or baby is too young to tell you what they need, look for signs from them. For instance, if you are cuddling them and they are pushing away, this may be a message that they are hot and don't want close contact, or if they are following you around and asking to be carried, this may be a message that they need close contact or comforting. Also, if they don't want to drink but are sucking their fingers, it may be that they need to suck on an ice block or a damp cloth to get small amounts of fluid.

There are five ways we, as practitioners and mothers, like to treat a child with fever. We love using Tissue Salts, Herbs, Homeopathic Remedies, Vitamins and healing foods.

Let's look at the very first steps to take when your child has presented with a fever.

You, as a parent or carer, need to be able to differentiate when it is wise to simply watch and observe your child's overall condition, and when to act. This is important because if you start to fuss and feel fearful that your child is getting sick, your child will pick up on your fear and will become fearful as well. Anxiety puts the body into a state of resistance and will slow down the body's ability to heal.

There are several questions you need to consider:

- Are they eating and drinking?
- Are they happy playing?
- Are they overheated?
- Are they whingy or whiny?
- Are they obviously unwell?

If your child's temperature is under 37.5° C, you can really just observe, taking into account the above physical conditions. If and when the temperature starts to rise and the child's behaviour changes, then jump in and start giving them the support outlined below.

Remembering you don't want to stop the fever, just support the body as it heals.

CHAPTER 10

Tissue Salts

Tissue Salts are also known as Cell Salts or Biochemical Minerals. They are regulators and restorers of body function, as they help the body absorb and distribute fluids and nutrients. Tissue Salts are an important first line of defence for children when illness or fever presents.

Tissue Salts provide the body with the minerals required to support the biochemical functions within the body, assisting the body's ability to recover. Given in the early stages of fever or illness, Tissue Salts will often prevent the process from deteriorating to later stages of infection or inflammation.

One of the first 'go to' remedies we personally and professionally use are Tissue Salts. These wonderful little remedies can often stop a fever in a few doses. This has been proven over and over again as patients report back to us.

Every one of your trillion or so cells have these salts in them. Tissue Salts are also called Biochemic Minerals because they are made from the exact mineral chemical pairings that the body uses. They were chosen as remedies because these minerals were found by Dr Schuessler (Med.) in 1872 to be the key mineral constituents of the body. Since then, his findings have been verified and confirmed by Depke and others.

Tissue Salts are formulated in the exact combination of minerals that your body uses to perform every task every day of your life from conception to death. A complete value of salts keeps your body's metabolism and homeostasis balanced as required for repair, health and survival. They are the building blocks to vibrant health.

In our current world of processed foods, chemically laden air and water, and a barrage of chemical medications we consume, we have allowed our body to suffer and become imbalanced in so many ways.

One of the very basic and most important measures you can take to rebalance your child is to know how to use Tissue Salts. Any health issue can be helped with these little gems.

There are 12 Tissue Salts that we routinely use:

- No 1 Calcium Fluoride - elasticity
- No 2 Calcium Phosphate - bones and teeth
- No 3 Ferrum Phosphate - first aid
- No 4 Kali Chloride - to support mucous membrane
- No 5 Kali Phosphate - stress, nerves and mind
- No 6 Kali Sulphate - chronic inflammation
- No 7 Magnesium Phosphate - muscle cramps and pains
- No 8 Natrum Chloride - the fluid balance salt
- No 9 Natrum Phosphate - the acid balance salt
- No 10 Natrum Sulphate - the excretion salt
- No 11 Silicea - the skin, hair and nails salt
- No 12 Calcium Sulphate - the blood-cleansing salt

Tissue Salt's job in the body is often summarised like this, each Tissue Salt has a whole range of functions. Your practitioner is trained in all of the different ways that your body uses Tissue Salts, how to recognise both acute and chronic mineral deficiencies, and Facial Diagnosis for signs and symptoms.

Tissue Salts Summarised

Authors Note: Depending on where you live, Tissue Salts may be known by other names, for example, Kali Muriaticum is called Kali Chloratum. These are the same Salts, just a different way of naming the Chloride salts.

Kali refers to Potassium salts, and Natrum refers to Sodium Salts. Each of these names may be used interchangeably.

We have used the German numbering system above. If you live in the United States, the Tissue Salts may be numbered differently with number 3 being Calc Sulph (Calcium Sulphate). So, if you read further about Tissue Salts, All German-based BBD approved publications use Schuessler numbering. However other publications may use either. You will need to check which numbering system they are using or you may not get the results you expect.

The numbering used in this book is the original numbering System used by Dr Schuessler and is still used in all the Biochemischer Bund Deutschland e.V. (BBD) based publications today. They are still the foremost researchers and knowledge base of the Works and use of the Biochemical Minerals of Dr Schuessler.

No 1 Calcium Fluoride (Calc Fluor)

Calcium Fluoride is known as the Elasticity salt. It helps when tissues are too hard, too elastic or too relaxed. It helps with conditions like muscular and ligament sprains and strains, dilated blood vessels like haemorrhoids and varicose veins and sluggish circulation. It's essential for the healthy development of bone surfaces and tooth enamel. It helps with cracked skin, and to soften hardened tissues in the body.

No 2 Calcium Phosphate (Calc Phos)

Calcium phosphate is the key building block of cells, and an essential mineral for building bone, teeth, bone marrow and connective tissues. Calcium phosphate is needed for binding blood proteins and is a clotting factor in blood and helps build up blood corpuscles. It is necessary for digestion and assimilation of foods. It is essential for all stages of growth, from baby's development in the womb, children's growth, recovery from illness, obstinate illnesses, and ailments in the elderly.

No 3 Ferrum Phos (Ferr Phos)

Ferrum Phos is the Oxygen Carrier of the Body, so helps with fever and inflammation, and is useful at the first stage of all illnesses as it brings oxygen to the tissues to provide the resources needed to fight inflammation. It is a vital component of the cells of all muscles, the brain, the liver (which is the organ containing the most blood), the intestine wall, and the villi of the small intestine. It is also a major component of haemoglobin. It has an important part to play in numerous enzyme processes in your body, and is also important, along with Vitamin C, for the structural integrity of cells.

No 4 Potassium Chloride (Kali Mur)

Kali Chlor is a key remedy for the second stage of inflammation when there are white discharges, mucous congestion and sinusitis. It helps ease respiratory disorders such as wheezing and chestiness, and swollen glands, sore throat, tonsillitis and middle ear infection. It activates the lymphatic system to process toxins ready for removal.

No 5 Potassium Phosphate (Kali Phos)

Kali Phos is essential for nerve and brain cells and for effective nervous system function. It assists with mental, emotional and physical exhaustion, including jetlag and the tiredness of shift workers. It's indicated when prolonged stress and tension cause nervous symptoms,feelings of anxiety and fear. It soothes nervous headaches, lack of energy, skin ailments, sleeplessness (including when the mind won't switch off) depression, nervousness, timidity, tantrums and bullying. This salt assists and calms all ailments of the nerves and mind.

No 6 Potassium Sulphate (Kali Sulph)

Potassium Sulphate is needed for chronic inflammation and is often used along with Ferrum Phos and Kali Chlor if the condition at the end of a cold is more chronic or developed to yellowish or greenish discharges. It is useful for disorders of the skin and scalp with scaling. It works in conjunction with Ferrum Phos, as an oxygen carrier to help respiratory, circulatory conditions and muscular aches and pains. It helps with intestinal disorders and 'liverish' conditions. It opens the pores of the skin, bringing blood to the surface and promotes perspiration. For this reason, it's useful when used in alteration with Ferrum Phos for fever, when the temperature rises in the evening.

No 7 Magnesium Phosphate (Mag Phos)

Mag Phos is essential for the muscles, and along with Ferrum Phos it helps muscular aches and pains, cramps, injury recovery and function. Mag Phos is essential for digestion, activating over 300 enzymes in the body. It is also essential for the nervous system, regulating the Autonomic nervous system, and together with Kali Phos to regulate both halves of the nervous system. It helps treat muscular cramps, spasms and minor nerve problems. It helps with spasm and pain of all kinds, like colic, menstrual cramps, palpitations, spasmodic croup, toothache, neuralgia. It's also helpful for exhaustion from emotional upset. It should be taken 2 hours away from time release medications as it can increase the body's speed of absorbing these medications.

No 8 Sodium Chloride (Nat Mur/Nat Chlor)

Sodium Chloride is needed to distribute fluids and regulate the amount of fluid in the tissues and help with the process of detoxification. Nat Chor is responsible for the manufacture and maintenance of mucus, so it's needed where there is too much fluid, like a clear drippy nose, or when tissues are dry, e.g. dry mucous membranes, which can lead to loss of taste or smell. It helps with some cases of constipation, backache, sunstroke, hay fever, and weak eyes, heartburn and digestive issues from too little acid. There may be a craving for salt or salty foods indicating that even if you are eating salt, the nutrition may not be getting into the cells.

No 9 Sodium Phosphate (Nat Phos)

Nat Phos attracts fluids to the cells. Without Nat Phos Nat Chlor can't distribute and Nat Sulph can't excrete fluids. Nat Phos helps maintain the alkalinity of the blood, emulsifies fatty acids and keeps uric acid soluble in the blood. Therefore, it can help young children who have been fed too much sugar and are suffering from acid conditions. It relieves reflux, indigestion, colic, skin conditions like eczema, and worms. It helps with stiffness and swelling of the joints, acidic blood conditions, rheumatism, and lumbago.

No 10 Sodium Sulphate (Nat Sulph)

Sodium Sulphate helps balance the amount of water in the tissues, and if necessary, helps to eliminate excess fluid. It aids the liver, spleen and kidneys. It relieves biliousness, liver troubles, digestive upsets. It relieves fevers with chills. In humid climates it helps the lungs balance the uptake of the fluid from the air. It helps with influenza, humid asthma, malaria, liver ailments. The tongue may have a brownish greenish coating, there may be a bitter taste and there may be a greenish-yellow colouring around the nose and mouth.

No 11 Silicon Oxide (Silica)

Silica is a component of all connective tissues, skin, hair and nails and helps with related conditions. It is a biochemic cleanser and eliminator. It promotes suppuration (the release of pus or infectious substances from a wound or sore). It initiates the healing process by dispersing potentially harmful substances accumulating in skin eruptions, toxic blood conditions, abscess, boils etc. In the first stage of any swelling, Ferr Phos, and Kali Chlor should be given, but if these salts fail to resolve the process, Silica can help to ripen the abscess and promote its discharge. It aids smelly feet and armpits, pus formation, abscesses, boils, tonsillitis, ear infection, brittle nails, and stomach pains.

No 12 Calcium Sulphate (Calc Sulph)

Calcium Sulphate is known as a blood cleanser, it helps clear away non-functional decaying matter and all conditions arising from impurities in the blood. If this material stays dormant in the tissues or slowly decays it can damage the surrounding tissues. Once pus or infection has found a vent or opening to leave from, Calc Sulph helps to close the infection. It is beneficial for slow wound healing and the last stage of suppuration (closing a wound after discharge) like pimples, boils, carbuncles, ulcers and abscesses. It's also useful for sore throats, colds, congestive earache, and UTI's

There are another 15 Tissues Salts that we can call on for body support if needed, however the above 12 salts are mostly what is required to bring the body back into balance.

No. 21. Zincum Chloratum (Zinc Chlor)

Zinc Chlor is the key Supplementary Tissue Salts for fever and the immune system. As well as being an important mineral to strengthen the immune system it helps with skin problems and emotional ailments. Dr J. G Redemache, used Zinc for brain afflictions, toothache, eye infections, headache, earache and skin disease.

Whilst Zinc has been used by medical practitioners since Paracelsus in the 16th century, it has only been rediscovered by modern medicine in recent years.

KEY FEVER REMEDIES

Treat the symptoms and look for the cause.

Below are some ways to treat fever, but it is always important to look for the cause. Why is there a fever? Is it from a cold or flu, an inflammation or infection? Is it from an infection under a tooth or in the ear? Is it from a baby teething? Is it from a gastric upset? Is there any pain? Best results will always be from not treating the fever alone but treating the cause as well.

In the cases of fever from tooth or ear infection, cold and flu, there may also be a process of suppuration where the body tries to eliminate toxins through mucous membranes, and skin (sweat). In teething, gastric infections or urinary tract infections the body may eliminate toxins through the bowels or urination. All of these are normal processes as long as they do not continue for an extended length of time.

The object of using Tissue Salts is to provide the body with the minerals it needs, at the time that it needs them, to perform these functions as quickly and efficiently as possible, so it can return to normal function without damaging other tissues. It is important to keep drinking water when there is a fever, to prevent dehydration, and aid nutrition getting into the cells and for the removal of toxins from the cells.

As fever is often part of the inflammation and infection process, the key remedies for fever will often be used in conjunction with other inflammation remedies. As you will see below, fever is generally the first stage and is well treated with Ferrum Phos. High fevers are best treated with Kali Phos to help remove the decaying matter that the fever has killed off and help the body eliminate it and deal with it so that further toxicity doesn't occur.

ABOUT INFLAMMATION AND INFECTIONS

The typical characteristics of inflammation are redness, warmth, swelling and pain in the affected area as the body tries to treat the problem and activate its defences. Some examples are fever, coughs, colds, influenza.

Inflammation often correlates to any of the disease processes ending in '-itis'; tonsillitis, bronchitis, gastritis, otitis, (middle ear infection), arthritis, meningitis, etc.

There are Three Stages of Inflammation

1. First stage – the body recognises the problem so starts attacking it and killing the pathogen. This action alone will heat up the body.

2. Second Stage - the body collects up the dead matter, or "millieu' and takes it for processing. Symptoms become differentiated, you will notice the fever along with other symptoms presenting.
3. Third Stage - the body eliminates the rubbish.

The Tissue Salt Remedies for Fever Inflammation and Infection

Ferrum Phos - first stage of inflammation.

At the first sign of a fever, cough, cold or other infectious process, the body will raise its temperature to try to fight the invading pathogen. The body starts sending out its defence force to fight off the infection.

HOW IT WORKS

If the body doesn't have enough of the mineral Ferrum Phos to fight the infection, it's like going into battle with a handful of foot soldiers, with the promise of more to come, instead of taking the entire army in the first instance. The body runs out of resources, and the inflammatory process lingers longer and takes over as there aren't enough soldiers to fight it.

WHAT IT LOOKS LIKE

Often the face is red, with rosy cheeks that are warm to the touch, as the body heats up and starts to fight the infection. The eyes might be bloodshot. The fever may start as a lower fever and get up to about 38.5 deg C.

Examples: fever, earache, cold, tonsillitis

Kali Chlor - Second stage of Inflammation

HOW IT WORKS

Once the body has started the immune response, it needs

somewhere to get rid of the rubbish, so it starts to gather it together in the lymphatic system ready to get rid of it.

WHAT IT LOOKS LIKE

The face is pale often with a bluish hue to the skin, there are often bluish purplish colourings around the eyes.

There can still be fever at this stage, with a pale face and lethargy.

Kali Sulph - Third stage of inflammation

HOW IT WORKS

Excreting the inflammatory material – time to clean out the garbage. This is often the yellow mucous snotty stage, as the toxins that have been gathered are excreted from the body.

WHAT IT LOOKS LIKE

You may see crusting yellowish snotty mucous coming out of the nose, sometimes you may see the skin show a yellowish triangle shape around the nose and mouth or a yellowish colour to the overall face colouring.

Kali Phos - High fever – Fever over 38.5 °C

HOW IT WORKS

When there is a high fever, the body gets exhausted if there isn't a supply of Kali Phos. The person gets lethargic, or a child may get floppy and want to lie down or sleep. Kali Phos helps them recover from this physically (and mentally) exhausted state.

Kali Phos also acts as an antiseptic. It processes the toxins of fever so that your child can recover faster. If the body doesn't have enough of this mineral the toxins stay in the body longer, decaying, and can prolong the fever (which we don't want, we want them out of the body so new cells can replace them).

WHAT IT LOOKS LIKE

Lethargic, tired, mentally emotionally and physically exhausted. Babies or children could be floppy or want to lie down, without much energy.

This is the type of fever that leaves you wanting to lie on the bed or on couch because there is nothing else you can do. There may be a greyish colour to the face.

Kali Sulph - Fever in late afternoon or evening

HOW IT WORKS

Kali Sulph opens the pores of the skin, bringing blood to the surface and promotes perspiration. For this reason it's useful when used in alternation with Ferrum Phos for fever, when the temperature rises in the evening.

Kali Sulph also supports the 'yellow systems' of the body, Liver, Gallbladder and Kidney, so helps with elimination of the toxins of infection.

WHAT IT LOOKS LIKE

The fever or any other associated symptoms come on in the late afternoon or evening. The child starts to sweat, or feel unwell. There may be a yellowish tone to the skin particularly around the nose and mouth.

Nat Sulph - Fever with chills

HOW IT WORKS

Nat Sulph helps to eliminate fluid from the body. In fever, the body loses fluids, often quickly. The body may dehydrate and not have enough fluids for the cells to function effectively. Hence the cells go into shock or cool down too quickly leading to chills or shuddering.

WHAT IT LOOKS LIKE

The patient is shivering and wants more blankets to warm up. Sweating may alternate between feeling chilly then feeling too hot and throwing off the blankets. Keep the patient warm and covered, give fluids, but also give 5 tablets of Nat Sulph which will help to rehydrate the tissues.

Nat Sulph also helps with chills and fevers in the tropics and subtropical climates where there is a large amount of humidity in the air. The body has difficulty processing the large amount of water molecules, so in turn suffers chills. Nat Sulph helps with the intermittent fevers of malaria, so is a useful remedy to have on hand in tropical climates. Nat Sulph helps the body to eliminate the excess water molecules breathed in from the humid air, and helps alleviate dehydration.

> "To speak from a chemical view, one molecule of Sodium Sulphate has the power to take up and carry out of the organism two molecules of water". *Dr W. H. Schuessler MD "The Clinical Science of Biochemic Medicine"*

Silica - Fever with teething, toothache, or earache

HOW IT WORKS

Fever in this case may be caused by an infection under the tooth or a build-up of infectious substances in the eustachian tube between nose/ mouth and ear. Silica helps to draw out infection under a tooth or in the eustachian tube. When children are teething, the teeth are trying to push through the gums. Silica helps the teeth to break through the gum or draw out an infection. If there is a discharge after giving silica, don't be concerned as it is a sign that the body has found a way for the infectious material to be released. It means it is working.

WHAT IT LOOKS LIKE

If your child has a fever with ear pain, mucous may have built up in the ear canal changing the pressure behind the eardrum and causing pain. They may be holding the affected part, want comforting, want to be held, or be restless and not want to be touched.

If your child is teething, the gums may get red and swollen, with or without the points of teeth being seen. In a tooth infection, the tooth may be sensitive or pain may travel into the gum or jaw.

In addition to Silica, in fever from toothache and earache, Ferrum Phos is often needed as the first remedy, and Mag Phos may be needed to help reduce pain, and calm the child. Don't forget to give yourself some Mag Phos and Kali Phos to calm you as well.

Mag Phos - Fever with Pain

HOW IT WORKS

Mag Phos helps to calm the nervous system and reduce pain and spasm. It is important to find what is causing the pain and address the cause.

WHAT IT LOOKS LIKE

The patient may be holding a part of their body, be restless or very still. Use the appropriate remedies to reduce the fever and use Mag Phos to help with the pain.

Their face may be very pinkish/carmine red with large blushing marks on the cheeks. Unlike Ferrum Phos, the cheeks are not warm/hot to touch. This redness may also appear during or after sport or exercise.

Please Note: If you can't work out the cause of the pain, or it is too severe, then seek appropriate treatment. In the meantime, Mag Phos will help to alleviate pain, calm the patient, and won't interact with other medications that may be given if required.

Nat Chlor - Fever with shivering

HOW IT WORKS

When there is shivering the need for Nat Chlor increases. Nat Chlor helps to distribute the fluids in and out of the cells, for toxins to be eliminated from the cells and nutrients to enter the cells.

Shivering is a process of rapid muscular contraction and relaxation used by the body to warm up the body to reach a temperature high enough to fight the infection.

Once the body reaches its new temperature "set point" the shivering stops. Shivering also helps warm areas that are cold and helps to distribute the heat to these areas.

Fevers can be felt through the whole body, or be localised to one hot area, for example, a hot head, and cold extremities. Nat Chlor works in tandem with the nervous system supporting the physical action of shivering to produce cellular energy and as a process to facilitate the exchange of nutrients and toxins in and out of the cell.

WHAT IT LOOKS LIKE

Even though the patient is hot to touch, they may be cold and shivering and wanting more blankets on. If the fever has produced a sweat this will cool the body temperature. The body may shiver to raise it again to the required temperature to fight the infection.

Nat Phos- Fever with acidic sweat

HOW IT WORKS

Nat Phos is needed to regulate the acidity of the tissues. One of the ways the body eliminates toxins, fats and excess acidity is through the skin via perspiration.

WHAT IT LOOKS LIKE

The child may be sweaty, or their skin may have a greasy or fatty shine to it.

The sweat leaves yellowish stains on clothes, particularly armpits of shirts, on sheets, and may cause a redness in the creases of the body where skin touches skin from the excess acid being eliminated through the skin. The child may have an acid mucous trail on their skin, for example a runny nose that leaves a red mark or trail on their face below the nostril.

The areas that are perspiring may have an underlying shine or matt appearance which may help determine the appropriate Tissue Salt to give your child.

For a simple way to differentiate which salt is required, simply rub a finger over an area of perspiration. If you use a finger to wipe the area of the skin that is shiny, and the shiny texture disappears, then Nat Phos is required.

If the shiny appearance remains after wiping the skin, then Nat Chlor is required.

Sweating may cause the skin to have a fatty shine that wipes off or changes to a matt tone if wiped with a finger.

Calc Phos - Recovery after Fever

HOW IT WORKS

Calc Phos is required for every function of the body. It is needed in convalescence after illness for the blood and all cells.

WHAT IT LOOKS LIKE

After a fever there is often lethargy and recovery time. Calc Phos is the key mineral needed to rebuild cells and aid recovery.

The child may be quite picky about what they feel like eating and need easy to digest foods because their digestive system isn't ready for heavier foods like red meat that take a lot of energy to digest, although they may be able to tolerate chicken or fish.

Fever with Convulsions - Seek Medical Attention

Febrile Convulsions generally are not life threatening. However, they may have medical causes beyond the scope of this book. It is important that you seek appropriate medical attention if you are concerned and remain calm.

Book an appointment with your doctor as soon as possible for a checkup if

- this is your child's first convulsion and you are concerned
- your child has never had one before AND it lasts longer than 5 minutes
- your child is very ill, won't wake up or looks very sick when the convulsion is over.

It is important to have the cause diagnosed. Knowing the cause will determine appropriate treatment.

A number of minerals may help address symptoms if your child has a convulsion:

NO 3 FERRUM PHOS

Helps manage the fever and provides the body with the minerals required to fight any infection.

NO 5 KALI PHOS

If the convulsions are due to an infection, Kali Phos will remove the toxins that may have triggered the convulsions.

NO 9 SODIUM PHOS

Helps remove excess acidity from the body, helping to attract fluid to the cells to rehydrate cells and flush toxins reducing the risk of convulsions.

NO 2 CALC PHOS

Helps the body to recover and relaxes the nervous system.

NO 7 MAG PHOS

Helps to regulate the nervous system, regardless of the cause of the convulsions.

How to Use Tissue Salts

Tissue Salt tablets dissolve in the mouth, are easy to take, and a great addition to your home medicine chest. The added bonus is that kids love them.

Please Note: the brands we use as practitioners dissolve in the mouth easily, allowing us to use them in lots of different ways: as compresses, as drinks, as pastes and powders. However, some of the brands found in health food shops can come in tablets that are much harder and require chewing or crushing or grinding first to be used in the same manner.

Tissue Salts are:

- Non-alcohol based
- Safe and easy to take – can be used during pregnancy
- Tasteless – particularly for children (and adults too)
- Fast acting – easily absorbed by the body into the bloodstream via the buccal mucosa (mucous lining inside your cheeks and floor of the mouth) so they can go straight to where they are needed. It doesn't matter if you have a "leaky gut" or other digestive issues because the body absorbs them straight into the bloodstream.
- Versatile – each salt has numerous uses in the body for every first aid or acute health scenario. It can even be taken for those in palliative care.
- Versatile - each salt has numerous actions in the body, and with an application for every first aid or acute health scenario.

There are numerous ways to use Tissue Salts

- take as tablets
- dissolve them in your water bottle for sport or exercise
- dissolve the tablets in a little water to give to babies on a teaspoon, or in a syringe tube by mouth
- crush them to use on certain wounds
- create a paste
- dissolve the tablets in water to use as a compress

Tissue Salt creams are also available in many countries for direct skin applications.

CHAPTER 11

Herbal Remedies

As herbalists, we rely on herbs a lot. We both love to grow them in our gardens and we both make our own teas and remedies. However, it is not necessary for everyone to do this as most herbs are easily available either dried, in tablet or capsule form, or as a liquid tincture. From your practitioner you can get an individualised, targeted herbal remedy made specifically for your situation.

Despite the common belief that herbs are not pleasant to take and children will reject them, it is not based in fact. One of the great advantages of herbal medicine is in its versatility to be presented to children in a variety of forms. From soothing herbal teas to delicious syrups or even herbal-infused ice treats or candied sweets and jubes, making them not only enjoyable for children to consume, but also a favourite.

Herbs, with their diverse range of medicinal properties, have long been recognised for their effectiveness in treating various illnesses. Herbs have been used for thousands of years and are the very first healing methods recorded. From China and India there are records of herbal remedies dating back over 5,000 years and have continued over the centuries to be used as a recognised primary form of health care. It is only in the last 100 or so years that drug therapy has taken the place of herbal medicine in mainstream medicine in the west. It was only 1938 when pharmacists in Australia were banned from making herbal preparations. In the last 10 years we have seen a resurgence of compounding pharmacies now making natural remedies again.

There is a herb for every ailment you can think of with each herb having a specific signature or uses related to its own unique family of actions on specific symptoms and illnesses. Whilst there is no "One Herb Fits All", herbs can be a very effective support for any illness and have been successfully used for centuries in every culture around the world. We have an excellent documented history of their value and use. Ancient Chinese, Ayurvedic, Native American, Australian Aboriginal and European herbal systems are just a few examples of the rich herbal traditions that have flourished throughout time and have relied on the power of herbs to alleviate ailments and promote wellbeing for their people.

Herbs have a wonderfully dynamic healing effect on the human body. They are very complex in their actions.

Although scientists have isolated and used some major active ingredients or constituents from many herbs, the resulting singled out ingredient has a limited range of actions, because isolating specific active ingredients limits the availability to the full spectrum of the chemistry within the plant. Herbal Medicine uses the whole plant giving access to the full spectrum of interactions of the herbal chemistry of each plant, that provides the plants unique form of "magic" when given as a Herbal Remedy. Herbal Medicine requires all the plant's complexity of active constituents to work synergistically in our very complex human body. And work they do!

Today herbs are becoming more valued as our resistance to antibiotics is increasing, and there is less time that we can use each antibiotic before it loses its efficacy. Also, bugs (infectious organisms) are becoming increasingly resistant to the vast array of available drugs. Herbs are so complex that the bugs don't become resistant to them. What a Godsend!

Medically, it is important to know whether an infection is viral or bacterial because antibiotics only treat bacterial infections and generally viral infections are left to run their course without medication. However, Herbal Medicine has herbs which treat bacterial, viral and fungal infections meaning that there is always a herb to support your symptoms regardless of what type of infection it is.

When your child presents with a fever, there are a variety of wonderful natural remedies you can choose from or combine together to support your child's healing. Herbal Remedies are ideal to treat *an infection*, in conjunction with treating the fever. The body has increased its temperature to activate all its innate healing mechanisms, enhancing the immune system's effectiveness, so it is natural to assume there is some form of infection in the body, and when you support the natural actions of the body, you are helping the body to do its job.

A Herbal Remedy as a tea or a tincture can contain herbs such as Echinacea, Yarrow, Ginger, Elderberry, Peppermint or Chamomile. In the initial stages of a fever, it doesn't matter that you don't know the name of the infection your child is fighting, just presume that they are fighting something, and treat the symptoms. Do all you can to support the fever process, and enhance the healing action, without interfering with the body's own healing mechanism. The action of the herbs won't stop the fever, and we don't want this. Herbs will help the body manage the fever, allow it to perspire, support the body's removal of the pathogens and any leftover debris or toxins, and then help the body cool down naturally.

There are a few considerations when giving herbs to children. You need to consider

- their age
- their weight
- how alert, sleepy, or responsive they are.

Remember, smaller doses given more frequently will give a gentle and efficient result. Some herbs can be taken at the child's appropriate dosage every half hour until the fever and symptoms are down to a manageable level.

Herbal teas are easy to give to children as they can be sweetened with honey to their taste buds delight! And of course, with the liquid consumed, they remain well hydrated which is vital when running a fever.

Herbal Icy Poles

Herbal teas can be frozen into Icy poles that children can suck on when they have a fever or feeling unwell.

Herbal Dosage Chart for Children

HERBAL TEA When the adult dose is 1 cup:	
Herbal Teas Age	**Herbal Teas Dosage**
Under 2 years	½ to 1 tablespoon
2 to 4 years	2 tablespoons
4 to 7 years	¼ cup
7 to 11 years	½ cup
Over 12 years	they can take the adult dose of 1 cup

Herbal Tinctures

There are several ways to use herbs. Robyn was trained to use drop doses which trigger the body's healing response and Molly was trained using both drop dosage and adult teaspoon/ml dosage. Molly uses both drop therapy and ml dosage depending on the situation, the ultimate aim is to provide a gentle pathway to healing. As practitioners, each patient is treated according to their body requirements, and their body strength, and the degree of illness presenting.

For your purposes, the chart below is a good guide for the maximum amount of a Herbal tincture to be used.

When the adult Drop-dose is 10-20 drops daily	
Herbal tincture Age	**Herbal tincture Dosage**
Under 3 months	See a practitioner
3 to 6 months	See a practitioner
6 to 9 months	2 drops
9 to 12 months	2 drops
12 to 18 months	2 drops
18 to 24 months	3 drops
2 to 3 years	3 drops
3 to 4 years	3 - 4 drops
4 to 6 years	4 - 6 drops
6 to 9 years	4 - 8 drops
9 to 12 years	5 -10 drops

For elderly patients, depending on their physical condition, usually 3 to 5 drops are sufficient.

Over 12 years they can take the adult dose per day or as prescribed by your herbalist. Depending on the circumstances the dosage may be administered up to 3 to 6 times a day.

Babies under 6 months of age, when breast fed, the mum can take the remedy. If not breastfed, the remedy needs to be put into 1 teaspoon of boiling water and cooled.

Babies under 6 months of age, please talk to your health professional before self-administering any remedies.

When the adult teaspoon dose is 1 teaspoon daily, continue to use drops for children, and consider the illness and their inner strength and capacity for using the higher doses.

Using Herbal Remedies

Let's look at some of the herbs used to support the body when in a fevered state:

Echinacea, Yarrow, Sage, Ginger, Elderberry, Peppermint, Chamomile

ECHINACEA

Echinacea is one of the most thoroughly researched herbs for fending off any infections, and in particular colds and flus.

Echinacea is well known for its ability to boost the immune system, making it an excellent natural remedy for preventing and treating any form of infection. From an immune supporting perspective, one of Echinaceas primary roles is in stimulating the production of white blood cells, which play a crucial role in identifying and fighting off any bugs. A lesser-known role of Echinacea is in its remarkable ability to help the body reduce fever as it kills off the offending bugs. One of its many functions in the human body is to act as a diaphoretic, inducing sweating, helping the body eliminate toxins and waste through the perspiration, assisting the body to heal, which facilitates a quicker recovery.

By encouraging the child's body to sweat, expelling not only excess heat but also harmful waste products produced by the bugs as they die off, Echinacea helps restore the body's balance as it continues to heal. This comprehensive support helps ensure that the child's body can effectively manage and overcome future infections with a stronger and more robust immune response.

ELDERBERRY

Elderberry is a powerful natural remedy with numerous healing benefits for children's health. Its antioxidant, immune boosting, antiviral and anti-inflammatory properties make it a valuable addition to support children's wellbeing. Elderberry can strengthen the immune system and provide relief from cold and flu symptoms. Its antiviral activity is highly effective in inhibiting the replication of many viruses, in particular viruses responsible for respiratory infections. By preventing viral attachment to host cells, Elderberry helps to reduce the severity and duration of viral infections, providing relief of symptoms and supporting a shorter recovery time.

Elderberry contains potent antioxidants, in particular anthocyanins, which play a vital role in its fever reducing ability, helping the body to ease inflammation, which contributes to the reduction of fever. It also has diaphoretic properties and aids in supporting the body to sweat, releasing excess heat and toxins.

SAGE

Sage is a herb that has been treasured for centuries due to its numerous health benefits. While sage is commonly associated with culinary uses, its healing properties extend far beyond the kitchen.

Sage has antispasmodic, expectorant, diaphoretic and antimicrobial properties, making it a valuable natural remedy for respiratory issues such as coughs, congestion and infections. Sage is known for its mild stimulating diaphoretic properties. By encouraging the body to release excess heat through perspiration, it supports the body to regulate during a fever, particularly when the child is experiencing chills and shivering. As the body perspires, it eliminates toxins helping to restore balance once more. This common kitchen herb has been used for centuries as a natural remedy to promote perspiration, reducing levels of toxins, and assisting the body in its fever-reducing ability.

PEPPERMINT

Peppermint is another of our common kitchen herbs, and as such is so often overlooked as a healing herb. It has antimicrobial, anti-inflammatory, diaphoretic, decongestant and expectorant properties.

One of the greatest actions of Peppermint is in its ability to act as an exceptionally effective herbal remedy to address fevers yet at the same time it does not suppress nor interfere with the body's innate healing abilities.

It helps reduce fever mainly due to its menthol content, which encourages sweating, helping to cool the body, while the anti-inflammatory compounds in Peppermint help to calm and soothe the inflamed tissues.

YARROW

Another herb with excellent anti-inflammatory and anti-microbial properties. Yarrow is known as a diaphoretic, astringent, tonic, and stimulant herb. It has been used for centuries for a great variety of health issues. It is widely recognised for its effectiveness in relieving fevers along with its immune boosting properties. Yarrow acts as a diaphoretic which induces perspiration, helping the body to sweat which will help clear the body of debris and toxins as the body kills off the bugs. Sweating is so important in a fever. It is a way the body works to keep the core fever going, but allowing the body to cool down as well, as sweating cools the external body. Yarrow helps to regulate the body's internal temperature during any infection or inflammatory state, supporting the release of heat from the body, and at the same time, effectively aiding the immune system to fight off any infections.

One of the other beautiful things about Yarrow is it helps with recurring coughs and colds, so if your child is continually getting cold, flu or infection, or other bugs at daycare, for example, Yarrow will often break the pattern. So, if your child is on the sickness merry-go-round, consider adding Yarrow to their health regime.

GINGER

Ginger is probably in every kitchen the world over. Cherished not only in the culinary world but also in medicinal practices.

Medicinally, Ginger has a multitude of health benefits, and in relation to fever, it is known as a diaphoretic herb, renowned for its powerful effects of contributing to the body's natural heating and healing processes by promoting sweating, a vital mechanism for regulating body temperature and expelling toxins. When the body heats up, ginger has a cooling action in the body, helping to lower the core temperature, which in turn allows the immune system to function more effectively as it works to eliminate infection and inflammation in the body.

Ginger's potent anti-inflammatory components help to lower the intensity and duration of a fever.

One of Ginger's most notable attributes is its antipyretic effect. Antipyretic herbs are those that help to lower elevated body temperature. By encouraging sweating, Ginger aids in cooling the body and preventing excessive rises in temperature. This cooling action is particularly beneficial as it supports the body's efforts to return to a normal temperature, allowing the immune system to operate more efficiently. As the core body temperature is managed effectively, the immune system can focus on addressing the underlying causes of inflammation and fever, leading to a more streamlined healing process. The dual action of both cooling and sweating helps to ensure that the body's core temperature remains within a range that supports effective immune function and faster recovery, without any complications.

CHAMOMILE

Chamomile is a very popular herbal tea. It conjures up thoughts of relaxation, calming emotions and lessening anxiety. It is however, so much more! Chamomile's benefits extend far beyond its reputation as simply a herb for relaxation. Chamomile is a versatile herb with many actions. It has antibacterial, antiviral, anti-fungal, anti-inflammatory, antispasmodic, diaphoretic and sedative effects.

The benefits of this herb in relation to fever, is in its anti-inflammatory, diaphoretic and sedative effects. During a fever, the body's inflammatory response can cause further discomfort to an already challenged body. By calming inflammation, supporting the body to perspire and helping to alleviate pain and discomfort, Chamomile calms your child and supports sleep, making this herb a valuable addition to any healing regime.

CHAPTER 12

Homeopathic Remedies

Homeopathy is a wonderful modality. Developed by Dr Samuel Hahnemann over 230 years ago, this is a modality that has been growing in popularity for the last 200 years and is now quickly taking hold all over the world. As you may know, Homeopathy is used by the British Royal family, with King Charles being a big advocate of it. It's also used by well-known sports stars and actors, as well as millions of people the world over. Homeopathy is taking its place as a very important healing modality.

Homeopathy is now a major modality in India and some South American countries where normal medical attention is extremely expensive. Medical training in India often integrates Homeopathy as well as conventional medical training. There is some fabulous research coming out of India: Sankarin, the Joshi's and Narayani and the Banerji Protocols are revolutionising the use of Homeopathy worldwide. Consequently, in India, Homeopathic Remedies are used as the main remedies in many medical clinics for numerous ailments.

The remedies are safe for everyone, even newborn babies. Generally used in a dose of 6x or 30c and taken as 3 pills under the tongue.

For acute situations, like fever, take one dose of 3 pills every 10 to 15 minutes for 4-8 doses until symptoms start to diminish. They can be repeated 4 times hourly or 3 or 4 times a day for a few days afterwards if needed. You stop taking the remedy when the symptoms are resolved. If there has been no change when taking the chosen remedy, reassess the symptoms and change the remedy. This is when is it so valuable to have a 'Homeopathic Kit' available at home.

The correctly chosen remedy will act very quickly. You can self-treat with Homeopathic Remedies for minor first aid problems with great success, however if an issue won't resolve using the remedies you have at home, or for any chronic or deep-seated problems, you will need to see a homeopathic practitioner.

Using Homeopathic Remedies

Let's look at some of the most useful homeopathic remedies for fever:

- Aconite
- Belladonna
- Ferrum Phos
- Gelsemium
- Arsenicum
- Bryonia
- Chamomile
- Bellis perennis

Aconite

This remedy is useful in the early stages of any illness, particularly if your child had been out in the cold or wind and was feeling very chilled. For fever that comes on suddenly, this is the first remedy to give your child. Your child may also be irritable, restless and anxious. They crave cold drinks, they don't want to be covered with blankets, may be very restless, and may experience waves of chill alternating with heat. The child is usually worse in the evening and at night.

Belladonna

A fever strikes suddenly, causing the cheeks to turn bright red. Your child may present with a red flushed face and/or ears, the cheeks in particular are flushed. The head feels hot to touch, yet their hands and feet can feel cold. They are thirsty for a cold drink. Everything hurts and their head feels like a cast iron ball has hit it. All your child wants to do is to retreat into a dark, quiet, warm room with a glass of cold water, juice or lemonade.

Gelsemium

Gelsemium is best with surprise attacks, the child is well one moment then suddenly quite sick, lethargic, tired, or feeling a loss of energy. It can also be helpful in a slow onset of symptoms which have been brewing for some time. The fever can come and go, the child can be lethargic, feel weak and dizzy, and often look a bit 'droopy'. Their face may look purplish. It's useful if your child is experiencing the classic 'hot and then cold' fever and they complain their head feels full, and they have chills running up and down their spine. Their body feels tired and heavy and there is a general weakness and often some trembling, and they don't even want to drink anything. This remedy is at the top of the list when it comes to summer ailments.

Arsenicum

This is one of my favourite remedies, as its healing support is vast, having a notable action on almost every organ in the body. In fever, this remedy is called for when the body feels cold, yet the head is hot, they can experience body pains and weakness.

The head can feel heavy. The child will feel chilly and want to be well covered and warmed, yet may want the window ajar. The child will often feel anxious and restless, and feel thirsty for warm drinks. Often there will be no perspiration until towards the end stage of the fever. Arsenicum is also really useful for fevers with or followed by vomiting or diarrhoea whether caused by fever, food poisoning, gastro bug or something else.

Ferrum Phos

The fever comes on more gently, and is not as intense as the Belladonna or Aconite fever. The fever can come and go. There is flushing on the child's face, yet there can be an overall paleness on the forehead, around the eyes and the chin area. They can be moderately thirsty, and are usually quite alert. It is also useful when children are feeling hot after sport or other physical activities.

Bryonia

This remedy is indicated when the child has body aches and pains along with the fever. The child feels thirsty, their lips and mouth may feel dry, and their body feels cold to touch, despite having a fever. There can be dizziness with the fever. The child wants to lie down and not move as it is too painful. Unusually they may wish to lie on the painful side.

Chamomilla

Your child may feel hot in certain areas of the body yet cold in other areas. They can have one red cheek and the other is pale. Chills and heat alternate, they want to be covered, and can be quite clingy and wish to be held or carried. They are a bit whinge and will ask for something only to reject it when supplied. Quite contrary!

Bellis Perennis

Whilst not specifically a fever remedy, Bellis is really useful in cases of overheating whether due to exercise or fever, where the patient cools down too quickly either by drinking iced water, having a cold shower or bath or using other quick cooling methods. Bellis helps to regulate the body back to the appropriate temperature and reduces symptoms that suddenly arise from this over-fast cooling.

CHAPTER 13

Vitamins and Minerals

When your child has a fever, and is fighting off a bug, it is good to give them a few vitamins as a way to build their immune system and support all their body functions, from immune development, bone growth to cognitive development. Children's bodies are constantly growing and developing at a fast pace, and they need a good range of vitamins and minerals to support that growth.

When they are unwell, the need for nutrients is greater and by adding extra vitamins and minerals to your child's daily routine, you support their body requirements for added nutrition.

There is a lot of information available now and a number of studies have shown that taking zinc and vitamin C during an illness, especially a cold, can actually shorten its duration by as much as 50 percent. We can only vouch for what we see with our patients, and there are three stand out vitamins that work well in most cases of infection, which is more than likely the cause of the fever.

Using Vitamins and Minerals

Vitamin C
Vitamin A, Vitamin D and Cod Liver Oil
Zinc

Iron
Other important nutrients Multi Vitamin
Probiotics

Vitamin C

Probably one of the best-known vitamins, as well as one of the most often ingested vitamins. The human body can't manufacture vitamin C, so we have to rely on getting it from our diet, or from supplements.

The RDA or recommended daily allowance, is very low. 90mg a day for an adult. That may well be enough to stop rickets from developing, however when it comes to fighting off bugs, we do need more. A lot more!

Vitamin C is unstable and is easily destroyed by heat and light, and because it is unstable, it is not always possible to be sure exactly how much is absorbed from our dietary intake. Because it is water soluble, you can eat lots of high vitamin C foods and you won't overdose on it. The same can't be said for taking Vitamin C supplements, as many adults find once they reach around the 2000mg mark, they get a very upset tummy and loose stools. It won't cause harm, just an upset tummy and often very dark urine. What this indicates is that the excess Vitamin C is actually excreted and not absorbed. Children would not need this high dose. 500mg or less may be their limit. Start with a lower dose, and slowly increase the frequency, and see how they go.

Vitamin C supplementation does help the immune system. It certainly seems to have an effect on the duration and severity on any form of infection. Vitamin C is essential to help the body absorb iron.

Vitamin A, Vitamin D and Cod Liver Oil

Firstly, let's take a look at Vitamin A and Vitamin D. Both vitamins as well as Omega 3 Fatty Acids are found in Cod Liver Oil.

Vitamin A

Vitamin A plays a role in immune function, supporting the health of skin and mucus membranes which serves as the body's first line of defence against pathogens.

Vitamin A is also essential for vision and tissue repair. No wonder Grandma always said, 'eat your carrots and you will see better'. For children we both like to use Cod Liver Oil instead of a Vitamin A supplement.

Vitamin D

Most people know that Vitamin D is freely available from sun exposure. This is great in summer but certainly an issue in the cold, overcast winter months, when there are often days or weeks with very little sun available. While we only need about 10-30 minutes of sunlight several times a week to get enough Vitamin D, depending on your skin type and where you live. When children are ill, they may not be getting enough sunlight exposure to fullfill the additional need to fight and recover from infection.

This essential nutrient enhances the immune system's ability to fight off infections, so is a vital component for healing. By providing an adequate intake of Vitamin D you are also helping your child's body reduce inflammation, which further supports their recovery process.

Vitamin D supplements are readily available however we both prefer to use Cod Liver Oil for children, especially during the winter months.

Cod Liver Oil

Most people have heard about fish oils, and have heard about the value of Omega 3, 6, and 9 fatty acids. But nowadays less people know about Cod Liver Oil. The difference between other fish oils and Cod Liver Oil, is that vitamin A and vitamin D are found in the Cod Liver Oil, but not in other fish oils.

Omega 3 fats are a crucial part of cell membranes. They improve heart health, support mental health, decrease liver fat, support infant brain development, help people manage their weight and fight inflammation. The best sources of omega 3 are the oily fish.

Omega 6 fats are plant-based oils, like Evening Primrose and Borage, and mainly provide energy. Omega 6 fatty acids have shown benefits in treating chronic disease.

Omega 9 are non-essential fats that your body can produce, if you have a healthy diet. Omegas 6 and 9 are found in plant oils, nuts and seeds.

Cod Liver Oil is very high in Omega 3 fatty acids (EPA and DHA), and is unique in its high levels of Vitamin A, Vitamin D and Vitamin K. Vitamin D is very important for the function of the immune system, and to ward off viral and bacterial infections. Cod Liver Oil is an age-old remedy, and has been used for many decades, specifically to boost the immune system in winter. My (Molly) personal experience of Cod Liver Oil was as a child growing up in the early 1950's, having to take Cod Liver Oil every morning before school, and it tasted terrible. However, looking back over my childhood years, I was very healthy during winter whereas my friend that I use to walk to school with often seemed to be ill with a cold, and I would have to walk to school by myself.

Consequently, as a health practitioner I have always used Cod Liver Oil for any winter illness with children, and big children too! These days you can get it in capsule form, or as a liquid with flavouring, making it so much more palatable for children.

Zinc

Zinc is a vital mineral that is found in every cell of the body. Zinc helps to support our immune system health, and aids in the activation of T cells which destroy bacteria and viruses. It also aids in wound healing and stimulates the activity of at least 100 enzymes. A really valuable nutrient. Zinc can help to shorten the duration of a cold and is particularly effective if you get some zinc lozenges to suck.

Don't take any zinc on an empty stomach as it can make you feel quite nauseous. Always take with food.

Zinc is in the same category as calcium, in so much as it is often quite heavily advertised, and you can buy it over the counter, so there is no way of monitoring how much zinc someone is taking, and yes, you can overdose on zinc. Once your zinc levels are maximised, when you take a zinc lozenge or liquid, you can get a very bitter unpleasant taste in your mouth. Nature's way of letting you know you don't need any more. When you simply swallow capsules of zinc, you don't get this same warning message.

Zinc is available as a supplement and as one of the additional Tissue Salts. Many Naturopaths have changed to using Zinc Tissue Salt as it is more palatable and they are getting better results regulating Zinc levels with the Biochemic Mineral and have more compliance as there are no taste issues. Also, the Zinc Tissue Salt doesn't have to go through the digestion to be broken down, whereas taking a supplement you lose at least half of the full value of the nutrient. When taking the Tissue Salt you get the full value.

The RDA of zinc for an adult is 15mg for men and 12 mg for women and varying amounts for babies from 2mg a day up to and 10mg for a child. As we get older we are unable to absorb it as efficiently. Also, if you have a high fibre diet, your absorption of zinc can be affected. So, a fine balance is needed.

Zinc is vital in any form of infection, particularly a viral infection. A mild deficiency of zinc can make you more prone to infections.

Iron

Iron plays an essential part for children when they have a fever. It maintains their energy levels and supports their body's immune response. With illness and particularly a fever, iron is required to produce haemoglobin, which carries oxygen to tissues throughout the body. This helps prevent fatigue and ensure that all organs and tissues function efficiently as they work to fight illness and speed up the recovery process, reducing the duration of the fever. Giving your child sufficient iron can help maintain their strength and resilience during any fever or illness, promoting quicker healing and a return to full health. For children, we have both used Floradix Iron tonic and a herbal liquid and vitamin combination as they taste good and is a natural way to get Iron into your child, without any constipation issues (a common symptom with iron supplements).

Other Important Nutrients

Multi vitamin

It can be useful to take a good multivitamin when your child is ill especially if they aren't eating a healthy, varied and balanced diet. Sadly, most people don't get the full nutritional value from their diet anymore due to how much processed foods are eaten. In this case, taking a good multivitamin makes good sense. Go to your health food shop and you will be able to get a good brand with a good balance of vitamins. Remember you get what you pay for, so stay away from the cheaper brands. They are not necessarily your best choice.

Probiotics

Probiotics although not an essential nutrient for fever itself, are an important nutrient for recovery after fever, infection, illness or after taking antibiotics or other pharmaceutical medications.

Probiotics are an essential addition to help support the immune system, which we now know, is very closely linked to your gut health. The gut is home to approximately 70-80% of the body's immune cells. Probiotics help to stimulate the production of antibodies and other immune cells that work to protect the body from any harmful bugs. Because children's immune systems are still developing, probiotics provide an effective boost to help fight off any infections and illnesses. Taking probiotics regularly can reduce the frequency and severity of many common childhood illnesses, such as colds, flu, and ear infections.

CHAPTER 14

Healing Foods

Foods play a very important role in healing. Having a healthy and varied diet full of fruits and vegetables, proteins, carbohydrates and fats, is always important.

When there is illness in the family, you can add certain foods that will boost immunity and aid in the healing process.

Isn't there always some new superfood that will heal everything? In the Internet age, there seems to always be more information about specific foods becoming 'superfoods' that will seemingly heal everything. Don't believe everything you read! We suggest you disregard all the hype about superfoods and go back to basics with your diet. Lots of vegetables, a few pieces of fruit, good meats and fish and some breads, rice or pasta. Balance is what is required. Nowadays, by adding herbs in cooking, salads, and as herbal teas you have access to all the superfoods that help to heal your body.

Herbs have been superfoods for centuries. In the past, apothecarists, shamans, herbalists, and pharmacists were the holders of the "superpower" knowledge of plants. Today, your naturopath or herbalist can help you determine whether a specific food or herb is the best for you, as no plant will heal everything for everyone. Just like you and I, plants have different properties specific to different aspects of the body's function.

Carbohydrate foods often get a bad rap. However, you need your carbohydrates, and the good stodgy ones like bread, rice, pasta, white potatoes play a really very important part in balancing your body. Particularly in winter, the body needs the stodgy foods to help keep your core body temperature warm and to keep energy levels up. A little-known fact is that white potatoes also play an important role in facilitating the production of healthy gut bacteria and probiotic balance.

Most people aren't aware that white coloured foods are often high in calcium and are often used as the first foods after illness, or in convalescence. Bland foods are easier to digest and then later other foods are added as the patient recovers.

As long as you are including a good variety of protein, vegetables and fruit in your diet, you will cover your bases, and your child will be getting the nutrients they need.

USING FOOD AS MEDICINE

There are a few key foods that will support your child when sick with fever, in illness, and to recover from the ensuing illness. We have broken these foods into first stage of illness and recovery stage foods.

FIRST STAGE OF ILLNESS

A great place to start when your child gets a fever or becomes ill is with nourishing drinks and liquid foods. Soothing and cooling drinks, warm teas and soups, provide the nourishment that's needed, but the body doesn't need to use a lot of energy to digest them. The body usually only wants liquid or light foods at this time.

Garlic

Well known for its ability to fight infection as antibacterial and antiviral. It also helps the body to detoxify heavy metals. It also aids digestion. "A peculiarity about Garlic is that it does not indiscriminately kill bacteria but is selective in its action so that (unlike antibiotics) it tends to destroy foreign pathogens while supporting the positive flora of the intestine." (Matthew Wood "The Earthwise Herbal") Garlic can be used in many ways. An old wives tale that really does work is to rub garlic on the soles of the feet when you go to bed. This simple act can stop a cold in its tracks and bring the body back into balance. The facts of why or how this can work is unknown, however, it may be the sulphur in the garlic that works its magic and draws out the fever or pathogen.

Onion

Onions have antibacterial qualities and may help fight potentially dangerous bacteria including E.Coli, Staphylococcus Aureus, Cholera bacteria, Helicobacter Pylori and many other pathogens. Onion helps boost immunity and improves digestive health. It is high in sulphur so helps the body to eliminate pathogens and toxins. Onion soup and honeyed onions are a great way to get this healing food into your child. See our recipe section for delicious healing recipes!

Honey

Honey is known for its antibacterial and anti-fungal properties. It is anti-inflammatory and useful in upper respiratory infections. Honey is the only food that never goes off, even if becomes candied. It is a great addition to soothing and healing drinks.

Lemon

Lemons are a powerful healing fruit and contain high levels of Vitamin C. They have an alkalising effect on the body and help to balance the pH. They improve immune function helping the body fight off infections and reduce inflammation. Lemons aid in your ability to absorb iron from foods, which helps increase your immunity. Lemons are a great addition to hot drinks, ice blocks, soups and as a zesty garnish for foods.

Additional Note: Vitamin C is essential to help the body absorb iron. Foods high in Vitamin C like lemons, tomatoes and capsicum are best added to foods high in iron to increase absorption, for example:

- Tomatoes with liver or red meat
- Lemon juice or parsley on spinach or broccoli
- Parsley as a garnish on meat dishes.
- Gremolata (zested lemon and chopped parsley) on winter casseroles. See Osso Bucco recipe

Lemon Balm

Lemon Balm is a cooling herb and useful in fevers to help cool the body. Lemon Balm can be used as a refreshing water, tea or as a garnish on desserts.

Cucumber

Cucumber is a cooling and soothing food and is mostly comprised of water. It aids digestion, and helps feed beneficial gut bacteria, improving gut health. By adding it to water it promotes hydration.

RECOVERY FOODS

Recovery foods are foods that are either easy to digest or high in nutrition for a small amount of food. Add these when your child is recovering from illness.

Potatoes

Apart from being a great comfort food (especially those delicious hot chippies), potatoes have good amounts of many minerals and vitamins, and in particular B6, Potatoes, like many other vegetables, have a concentration of fibre, vitamins and minerals close to the skin, so do leave the skin on. Potatoes are important for the gut microbiome, and act like a prebiotic. Potatoes are great added to stews, soups and casseroles, mashed potatoes, and of course kids love homemade chips, wedges and potato skins.

Red capsicums

Red Capsicums have the highest value of vitamin C of all vegetables as well chilli or Cayenne pepper, which is added to our 'kick a germ' drink. These foods help to transport oxygen around the body, are super helpful in treating a fever and most importantly, they nourish the heart. Chilli also helps the body to sweat, causing a cooling effect. Red Capsicum can be cut into strips for finger foods, cut into squares for crudities with dips, added to stews, salads and rice dishes. Make char-grilled capsicum over a flame of high heat, or in the oven.

Acerola Cherries

This is an interesting cherry and not often considered by the home gardener. They are very high in vitamin C and are often compounded with Vitamin C in tablet form. It is a lovely tree to grow at home, and it grows well in pots. The cherries are smaller than the big cherries you are normally used to seeing in the fruit shop, and they are not perfectly round, but are misshapen and they taste a bit bitter initially, but once you get used to eating them they are delicious. The fresh cherries are great for the kids to snack on.

Papaya (Paw Paw)

Papaya is the one of the best fruits for vitamin C. Paw Paw along with Pineapple and Kiwi fruit have the highest proportion of enzymes to aid digestion. Fruit can be a refreshing snack when your child has a fever, or in a fruit salad or with yoghurt.

Parsley

This is the original superfood, high in iron. It helps regulate the fluid balance, is high in antioxidants, and a good source of Vitamins A, C and K. It has antibacterial properties and is helpful in fighting infection. It is easy to add as a garnish or ingredient into most foods, for its high nutritional value, flavour and decoration.

Bone Broth

Bone broth is made by boiling bones, often with other vegetables, to create a nutritious broth. The broth extracts nutrients from the bones, and vegetables and is high in many nutrients, including calcium. It is a great base for soups, casseroles and many other dishes. It is a highly nourishing addition to the diet when children are a bit off their food and can even be had as a drink.

Miso

Miso has gained popularity in the last few years. It is a nutrient rich food, which uses a fermentation process to extract the goodness that aids digestion, boosts the immune system and helps the body fight disease. The varieties made from soybeans contain all the essential amino acids needed for human health and are considered a source of complete protein. The fermentation process used to make Miso promotes the growth of natural prebiotics that are essential to healthy digestion, making it easier for the body to absorb the nutrients it contains. Miso makes nutritious soups or broths, can be consumed as a drink or as a soup base.

Junket

Junket is a little-known food which is easily made using junket tablets bought from the supermarket. Junket tablets are added to warmed milk making junket or what used to be called "curds and whey". Make a number of individual glasses, cups or bowls of junket, as a recovery snacks or desserts for your child. Junket is a forgotten food, that is not only good for health but tastes delicious too!

CHAPTER 15

Healing Protocols

TISSUE SALTS

When your child is first unwell, they will usually present with a mild fever, which is a fever up to 38.5°C. Their face may appear flushed with a large red circular spot on one or both cheeks, or they be red in the face. The skin may be warm to touch, and they may feel hot or chilled or alternate between both. They may be full of beans or they may be obviously lethargic and fatigued.

Remembering that fever helps to fight off the infection, and you don't want to bring the fever down, just support the body in what it needs to do.

PRESCRIPTION:

FIRST STAGE:

Supporting the body as it develops a fever.

Tissue Salts

1 x No 3 Ferrum Phos every 15 to 30 minutes
For High Fever, add
1 or 2 x No 5 Kali Phos, every 15-30 minutes

Giving the appropriate Tissue Salts over the first few hours, with or without the appropriate homeopathic remedies or herbal remedies, will often see most fevers resolve naturally in a few hours or overnight. As soon as you can, treat the cause or infection with herbs and homeopathic remedies, and most symptoms will usually be resolved within 24-48 hours. Any lingering symptoms will resolve over the next few days, if they haven't already.

Look for the Cause

Once you are satisfied the fever is stable, look for the cause of the fever.

- Is it from something they ate or drank? 2 x No. 3 Ferrum Phos, 2 x No. 4 Kali Chlor
- Do they have vomiting, reflux or diarrhoea with it? 2 x No. 9 Nat Phos, 2 x No. 2 meal, Calc Phos each meal
- Are they dehydrated or experiencing chills, or suffering sunstroke? 2 x No. 10 Nat Sulph hourly, 2 x No. 8 Nat Chlor each meal
- Have they been around someone who is sick or was sick recently? 2 x No. 3 Ferr Phos and 2 x No. 4 Kali Chlor every hour
- Do they have an ear infection, are teething or have a tooth infection? 2 x No. 11 Silica every hour
- Was it a windy day? This sounds like a silly question. But wind does have an effect on some people's nervous system. A windy day can overstimulate some people, just like too much noise or lights can overstimulate other people. Kids can get restless, pernickety, emotionally restless. 2 x No. 11 Silica, and 5 x No 6 Kali Sulph
- Have they had an emotional upset? Is there something that upset them that they have suppressed or pushed down or haven't been able to express properly? Have you noticed that

anger or shame can cause an increase of body temperature? This can feel or look like a fever, but may not last as long. If the feelings can be safely felt, expressed or experienced, and allowed to run their course, with the child feeling safe and comforted, the emotions can transform and the heat will often dissipate naturally. 5 x No. 7 Mag Phos is a good Tissue Salt to use to calm the nervous system, or when any questions you ask cause them to blush from embarrassment, shame or fear, causing emotional reactions. 5 x No. 3 Ferr Phos for overexcitement or overstimulation, (physical, mental or emotional). Their face is warm to touch, and they may look or feel feverish or be dizzy.

Notice how when you can work out what the cause of the fever is, you naturally start to calm down and become less fearful yourself. This is the start of empowering you. This gives you a focus to assess the situation and work out what to do next. You now have less reason to be fearful.

Note for Parents: To calm yourself when your child has a fever or any sudden acute illness, take 5 x No. 5 Kali Phos and 5 x No. 7 Mag Phos. This will help you to be calmer and the best support for your child no matter what happens next.

HOMEOPATHIC HELP

Low fever 38.5 deg or lower

Use whatever potency you have in your kit. 6x or 30c is most often used.

Ferrum Phos - Fevers come on slowly with temperature creeping up over a number of hours, with a pale face with circular flushing of the cheeks. Low fever. Especially helpful in fever due to ear infection. Useful for the very first stages of fever when you can't yet ascertain the cause.

Gelsemium - Fever comes on slowly, sometimes over several days. Purplish or purplish-blue colouration to the face. The child doesn't want to get out of bed, wants to lie down and doesn't want to move. They have a droopy appearance. It is particularly useful for fevers in summer, and when the fever is worse in the afternoon.

High fever 38.5 or higher

Aconite - Fever comes on quickly, often at 7pm or midnight. The child is restless in bed and may throw off the covers. The fever may come on after a windy day, being exposed to dry, cold air or getting a chill, after emotional upset, shock or trauma. Also useful for a fever due to a sudden infection.

Belladonna - Fever comes on quickly. The patient is very red faced or very pale. Belladonna can be helpful if the patient is in a lot of pain with high fever from earache.

The patient may be limp or listless, and not very responsive.

HERBAL HELP

From the first signs of fever, it is important to boost the immune function. In most cases of fever there will be a bug, viral or bacterial, involved. Often at this stage of fever, with a combination of a homeopathic remedy, a tissue salt and a herbal remedy, within 24 to 36 hours your child will have thrown off whatever it was they had contracted and be back to their normal bouncy selves.

Start with regular dosing of Echinacea or better yet the Kidz Immune Boost Tea (See Recipes section) that we have formulated specifically for children with fever. Give your child an age-appropriate dose.

VITAMIN SUPPLEMENTS

Give maximum amounts depending on the age and weight.

Vitamin C, Zinc and Cod liver oil, you can crush any tablets and make a bit of a 'vitamin toddy' in a juice or coconut water or anything to help your child get it all down.

Probiotic

Give your child a probiotic to aid the microbiome aid the balance.

FOOD HELP

Kidz Immune Boost Tea, Kick A Germ Drink or Kick A Germ Juice - see recipes and variations in Chapter 16. Choose the best combination for your child's situation, based on what you have in your pantry.

A bowl of homemade chicken soup would be ideal at this point.

A few healthy Gummies, see our recipe below.

Definitely no sugary lollies, candies or pop drinks. Stay away from commercially produced fruit juices.

Keep your child calm and relaxed. Even if they still want to run around, settle them down into a quieter, calmer state and perhaps read a book or let them watch their favourite TV show. The body's healing ability is exponentially increased as the body rests. The immune system works twice as fast when asleep than when you are awake. Rest and Heal!

SECOND STAGE

Dealing With The Inflammation

Often as the child moves into this stage, they are starting to feel a bit tired and will be willing to rest. As the body is well into the immune response, it is starting the process of gathering up the pathogens into the lymphatic system to clear the rubbish or toxic load.

What it physically looks like: The face is pale, often with a bluish hue to the skin. There are often bluish-purple colourings around the eyes.

TISSUE SALTS

Kali Chlor is the key Tissue Salt for the Second stage of Inflammation. Alternate Ferr Phos and Kali Chlor to provide the key nutrients to treat the second stage of inflammation.

Suggested Prescription:

1 x No. 3 Ferr Phos every hour (eg 1pm, 2pm. 3pm)
1 x No. 4 Kali Chlor every hour on the half hour (eg 1:30pm, 2:30pm, 3:30pm)

Whilst these two Tissue Salts are mentioned for the second stage of inflammation, we will often give both of these from the very start of the fever, as Kali Chlor will become depleted quite quickly after a fever starts.

If you have determined the cause or have noticed other symptoms, give the appropriate Tissue Salt as outlined in the Tissue Salts section. Usually, you can give 2 tablets every hour or two until symptoms diminish, then reduce frequency to 3 times daily until all symptoms clear completely. At this stage of development is important to add the herbal remedy and homeopathic remedies as appropriate. The immune system requires support to fight off the bugs.

HERBAL HELP

Keep giving regular doses of Kidz Immune Boost Tea or any of the recommended herbs that you have. Echinacea is particularly valuable, and of course, give the age appropriate dosage. As there is still fever, the body is still in its 'kill off' phase and working hard. You need to keep the support ongoing.

A good herbal combination for Stage Two is Echinacea, Elderberry and Ginger.

VITAMIN SUPPLEMENTS

Continue giving Vitamin C, Zinc and Cod liver oil. You could crush any tablets and make a bit of a 'vitamin toddy' in a juice or coconut water, anything to help your child get it all down.

Probiotic - give your child a probiotic one or two times a day.

FOOD

Often children will be off their food, so give hot teas or broths, and have a few gummies or frozen herbal icy poles (or ice treats) for them to suck on or to tempt them with. It is vital to keep fluids up.

THIRD STAGE

This stage deals with clearing debris and removing toxicity.

TISSUE SALTS

2 x No. 6 Kali Sulph 3 times daily. If there are any lingering symptoms, use any of the Tissue Salts needed that fit the specific symptoms.

HERBAL HELP

In this third stage of healing, continue to give the herbal remedy which contains the diaphoretic action that stimulate the body to perspire, and release the debris, which will support the body in its final healing phase and allow the fever to recede.

Continue to give your child our Kidz Fever Fighter Tea, or Echinacea or whatever you have at home. Give an age-appropriate dose. Sweeten it to taste with honey.

Yarrow if they have a recurring cough, cold or fever. Sage if they have a sore throat.

Chamomile if the child is particularly clingy, whingy and whiny and has changeable emotions.

A lovely combination for children could be Ginger, Chamomile, Peppermint and Elderberry, which would help the body to cleanse and heal.

VITAMIN SUPPLEMENTS

Continue to give maximum amounts for age and weight. Vitamin C, Zinc and Cod liver oil along with a Multi Vitamin. Continue with a Probiotic.

It is good to keep taking the vitamin supplements for 2 or 3 weeks after the fever and illness has abated, to bolster their immune system.

FOOD HELP

Lots of the nourishing broths, and soups. Start to introduce more solid foods like the chippies and snacks, and towards the end of the healing process slowly introduce heavier foods, like the Osso Bucco in our recipe section, or any favourite main meal, if they feel up to eating it.

They may just feel like toast. Offer some dips and veggie sticks. So long as they are eating, and keeping up their intake of fluids, they will recover quickly as this third stage comes to an end.

RECOVERY STAGE

During the next two to three weeks, it is beneficial to continue with a maintenance protocol to support the recovery of the immune function and to revitalise their system.

TISSUE SALTS

Continue taking 1 x No. 3 Ferrum Phos and 1 x No. 4 Kali Chlor each day for the next month. If your child has been suffering with a recurring illness, continue this protocol for the next three months, treating any acute situations with the prescribed protocols above. Doing this you will find that children will fully recover their health back to a healthy status quo.

HERBAL REMEDIES

Continue with Echinacea, at the child appropriate dose, for the entire winter months.

HOMEOPATHIC REMEDIES

Homeopathic remedies are only for acute situations and are not used as a preventative or for ongoing maintenance. If your child has recurring or ongoing symptoms, consult with your homeopath for a personalised prescription.

VITAMIN SUPPLEMENTS

Continue with the Vitamin C, Zinc and Cod Liver Oil throughout the winter months. Continue with a probiotic for at least a month after illness or any pharmaceutical medications.

FOODS

In the recovery weeks continue to give easily digested recovery foods and slowly introduce more robust foods as your child returns to normal. If your child's energy lags at any time, continue to add these soothing foods into your family's regular meal plan to boost everyone's health and immunity.

CHAPTER 16

Food for Health Recipes

Both Molly and Robyn have used food as medicine for a long time. Molly taught nutrition at NatureCare College for several years and kitchen tested lots of different recipes for herself and for her clients to assist with different dietary sensitivities and ailments. Molly's 'Magic Mix' is a winner, and kids will love her gummy recipe when they are sick.

Robyn loves food and cooking and has played with different recipes and flavours over the years. She knows first-hand what would work with her kids when they were sick. Onion soup, tuna casserole and hot drinks were always a favourite.

These recipes are chosen specifically because we have tried and tested them for adults but especially for children who can be quite picky. We also wanted to make sure that these recipes are easy for everyone, especially parents who may not have been taught how to properly feed their kids when they're feeling unwell.

What most parents don't know is that there are very easy solutions waiting for them in their kitchen. With a few, small, staple additions to your fridge or pantry, any of these recipes will become second nature to make. And once you and your kids have experienced the healing benefits of these foods and drinks, you will find that they will often ask for them the next time they are ill. Kids are very attuned to what their body needs.

Around 80% of our immune function is in our gut, so let's nourish and heal it as best we can with some really delicious and healthy foods that your kids will enjoy eating, even when they are feeling a bit off.

The following few recipes are simple to make and easy for kids to eat even when they have a sore throat. Which recipe will be your kids' favourites?

What Can You Feed Your Children When They Are Sick?

Many parents struggle with what to feed their children when they are sick. Children are often pickier when they feel unwell, and if asked will often prefer a snack to a meal. Parents will often give a packet of chips or some simple and easy to buy processed snacks, because it feels like an easy solution, and they know their child will probably eat it. What most parents don't know is that there are some easy solutions waiting for you in your kitchen. With a few small additions to your fridge or pantry items, any of these recipes are easy to do and once your children experience the healing benefits of these foods and drinks, you will find they will often ask for them the next time they are ill. Kids are very attuned to their body requirements.

Given that we have around 80% of our immune function in our gut, let's nourish and heal the gut with some really delicious and healthy foods your child will enjoy eating, even when they are feeling a bit off.

The following few recipes are simple to make, easy to heat up, and easy for kids to eat, even when they have a sore throat.

Kick a Germ Drink

You probably know about honey and lemon tea or honey, lemon, and ginger tea. Here are some great variations that I learnt from Dorothy Hall Herbalist, which she called "Kick a Germ Drink." These variations help anyone start to feel better.

Ingredients:

½ lemon, squeezed
1 garlic clove, crushed
1 tsp honey
½ cm cube fresh ginger, crushed, or ¼ tsp dried ginger
1 pinch to ¼ tsp cayenne pepper
Hot water

Instructions:

Put the squeezed lemon juice into your cup (at least 1 tbsp; add more if lemon is juicy). Optional: drop in the rind to infuse for added benefits. Add honey, garlic, and any combination of ingredients below. Pour hot water over and sip when hot, warm, or cool.

Variations:

1. Hot water, lemon, honey — good for any illness
2. Hot water, lemon, garlic, honey — use if you suspect infection
3. Hot water, lemon, garlic, honey, ginger — good for sore throats, coughs, colds. Soothing with or without garlic
4. Hot water, lemon, garlic, honey, cayenne pepper — strong germ-fighting combination that provides energy for healing

Notes:

- Suitable for children of all ages and adults at the first stage of fever, colds, sore throats.
- Babies under 2 years: allow to cool and give 1 tsp at a time using variation 1 or 2.

Kick a Germ Joy Juice

This is a honey-based herbal infusion with garlic, lemon, and yarrow, designed to gently support the immune system. Yarrow can be found at most health food stores.

Ingredients:

1-2 cloves garlic
Rind of half lemon
1 tsp Yarrow
3-4 tablespoons of honey to cover

Instructions:

Cover the herbs with honey in a jar and store in the fridge. To make a hot drink, add 1 tbsp of honey liquid to a cup of hot water.

Variations:

1. Hot water, garlic, lemon, honey — if yarrow is unavailable
2. Substitute yarrow for fresh or dried parsley, sage, or chamomile
3. Use a chamomile tea bag as a substitute for yarrow

Notes:

- Works as a daily tonic or at the first sign of illness.

Mmm… Molly's Magic Mix

Molly's Magic Mix is a yummy, hot, and powerful spoonful of immune support! It is delicious and can be taken as a tea.

Ingredients:

1 medium onion
2–4 garlic cloves (depending on taste)
3 cm piece of ginger
Juice of 1 lemon
Cayenne chilli (optional, depending on tolerance)
Honey to taste

Instructions:

Place all raw ingredients into a food processor and blend until smooth. Store in the fridge. Add ½–2 tsp of mixture to a cup of boiling water to drink as tea.

Notes:

- Quantity is flexible according to taste.
- Children may prefer a milder version.

Kidz Immune Boost Tea

This tea is a gentle herbal blend to support children's immune systems.

Ingredients:

2 parts echinacea
1 part olive leaf
2 parts elderberry
1 part calendula

Instructions:

Mix all dried herbs together and store in an airtight container. Use 1 rounded tsp per cup of boiling water. Cool to a safe temperature for children and sweeten with honey if over 12 months old. Take 3–4 times a day.

Notes:

- Herbs can be purchased individually and mixed.
- Adjust dosage by age and taste.

Kidz Fever Fighter Tea

A gentle tea to help reduce fevers and soothe symptoms.

Ingredients:

2 parts echinacea
2 parts lemon balm
1 part yarrow
1 part chamomile
½ part ginger
Honey to taste

Instructions:

Mix all herbs together and store in an airtight container. Use 1 rounded tsp per cup of boiling water. Cool for children and sweeten with honey if over 12 months old. Take 3–4 times a day. Sweeten with honey as needed.

Notes:

- Excellent for supporting the immune system during fevers.
- Health food stores have a great range of individually packed dried herbs. You can purchase the herbs, mix and store in an airtight container.

Fenugreek Tea

Fenugreek tea may not be the most delicious option, but it's highly effective at helping a fever resolve quickly and effectively. Commonly used in Indian cooking and valued for its cleansing properties, it supports the body's natural detox process. As it works, perspiration can become noticeably strong-smelling. This is a sign that toxins are being released.

For adults, it's best to drink Fenugreek tea on a weekend or while resting at home, when you're less likely to be in social settings. Avoid using anti-perspirants during this time and allow the body to sweat freely as part of the detoxification process. Though the scent may be stronger than usual, the fever often passes quicker and the body is able to cleanse itself naturally.

Ingredients:

1 tsp fenugreek seeds
1 cup hot water

Instructions:

Steep fenugreek seeds in hot water and sip several times throughout the day.

Notes:

- Perspiration may have a strong odour so best taken at home.
- Helps to naturally remove toxins.

Lemon, Cucumber, Lemon Balm, and Mint Water

These waters help cool fevers, regulate body temperature, and refresh children. They are equally refreshing on a hot summer's day as a drink by the pool, after sport or running around in the sun, after sunburn or even a sunstroke. Make up a jug and place it by the child's bed, in the fridge, on the table for everyone to grab a drink, or on your desk while working. The longer the ingredients sit in the water, the more the water infuses with the nutrients from them. A jug is a great way to keep track of exactly how much fluid your child is drinking.

Ingredients:

½ small cucumber, sliced
½ lemon, sliced or in chunks
3 sprigs lemon balm or mint
Water

Instructions:

Place ingredients in a large jug and fill with water. Allow to sit for 5 minutes before drinking.

Notes:

- Refreshing for summer, post-sport, sunburn, or sunstroke.
- Can add ice cubes.
- Combine one or multiple ingredients as desired.

Coconut Water

Have you tried drinking fresh coconut? Crack it open and pour out the water. It's absolutely delicious! Fresh coconut water is soothing and nutritious, supporting hydration and energy. Coconut is high in potassium, which is needed to fight infection, and provides energy when a fever has left you feeling lethargic. If you don't have access to fresh coconuts, coconut water is readily available from the supermarkets now-a-days.

Notes:

- Use young drinking coconuts with soft flesh, not the round, brown, dried ones.
- Add coconut flesh for added nutrition.
- Bottled coconut water works if fresh coconuts are unavailable.

Homemade Lemonade

Kids love lemonade. Sadly, when commercially made, it is full of sugar and not even slightly good for our body, especially when fighting off a bug. This recipe is a healthy, refreshing alternative to commercial lemonade that kids will eventually love!

Ingredients:

Juice of 4 lemons
3 cm fresh ginger
Soda water, mineral water, or coconut water
1 garlic clove (optional)
Honey, coconut sugar, or maple syrup to taste

Instructions:

Crush or blend ginger and garlic with lemon juice. Add honey to taste and mix thoroughly. Add 1–2 tsp of this cordial to a glass of soda, mineral, or coconut water.

Variations:

Basic lemonade without garlic and ginger

Notes:

- Adjust garlic and ginger to taste.
- kids may prefer a sweeter, milder version.

Healthy Gummies

These gummies or soft jubes are excellent for kids and adults. Quick and easy to make.

Ingredients (1 cup batch):

1 cup liquid (fruit juice, boiled herbal liquid, Kidz Immune Tea, or coconut water + 2 tsp grated ginger)
3–4 tbsp gelatin powder
Honey to taste

Instructions:

Stir honey into the liquid, then mix in gelatin. Sit 5 minutes until thickened. Cook gently over medium heat for 5 minutes, stirring constantly. Pour into silicone moulds. Freeze for 20 minutes (do not fully freeze). Store in the fridge.

Notes:

- Adjust gelatin for desired firmness: 4 tbsp for firm, 3 tbsp medium, 2 tbsp soft.
- Small batch: ⅓ cup liquid + 1–1½ tbsp gelatin + honey.
- High-acid fruits like pineapple may prevent setting.

Junket

Junket is a digestible milk dessert, often tolerated by children with milk sensitivities. Junket tablets are available in your supermarket, and they are made from rennet, which is an enzyme used in cheese making. It's quite likely that your child might never have tried junket. So, give it a whirl. It is simple but delicious!

Ingredients:

2 junket tablets
350 ml milk
Sugar to taste
Nutmeg, grated

Instructions:

Gently warm milk to body temperature. Dissolve junket tablets in a small amount of water. Stir into milk, pour into individual glasses and allow to set. Sprinkle with nutmeg.

Notes:

- Works best with full-cream milk (cow, goat, or sheep).
- Milk substitutes or skim milk may not set.
- Can help settle upset tummies.
- Milk should be the same temperature that you would use when heating a baby's bottle. Warm to touch, as you check it against your inside wrist.

Honeyed Onion Syrup

You are not going to believe how yummy and nutritious this is. We absolutely love this mixture! It sounds like something you would never consider trying but be prepared to be surprised. It is very soothing for sore throats, and the antimicrobial benefits of the onion supports any upper respiratory illness.

Ingredients:

1 large onion
Honey

Instructions:

Finely slice the onion and cover with honey in a bowl. Cover and refrigerate for a few hours or overnight. Take 1–2 tsp of the honeyed onion syrup every hour or two.

Notes:

- Purple onions are preferred but any variety works.
- Only drink the honey-infused liquid; do not eat the onion.

Raspberry Syrup

A versatile syrup for drinks, icy poles, or pancakes.

Ingredients:

200 g raspberries, fresh or frozen

½ cup coconut sugar

150 ml water

Instructions:

Cook ingredients over medium-high heat until simmering (about 10 minutes). Stir frequently and strain to remove seeds. Store in the fridge or freeze in ice cube trays.

Variations:

1. Icy poles: combine with milk, coconut milk, or yogurt
2. Ice blocks: mix with water
3. Syrup: use over pancakes, yogurt, or muesli

Notes:

- Adjust water ratio for thicker or thinner syrup.

Tapioca

Tapioca or sago is a delicious, soft, jelly-like dish.

Ingredients:

¼ cup tapioca pearls
1 cup milk (coconut or other milk of choice)
1 cup water
1 tbsp sugar, or to taste
½ tsp rose water or ½ tsp vanilla extract

Instructions:

Soak tapioca in water for a few minutes. Add remaining ingredients and bring to a boil. Stir continuously to prevent sticking. Simmer until pearls are transparent (about 15 minutes). Serve warm or cold; it will set like jelly when cold.

Berry Nice Yoghurt

A quick, fruity snack or breakfast.

Ingredients:

1 cup frozen berries (raspberries, blueberries, strawberries, or a combo)
1 cup yoghurt
3 dates, pitted
2 tsp honey

Instructions:

Blend dates, berries and honey until smooth. Stir in yoghurt and serve. Optional: freeze in icy pole containers.

Healthy Homemade Stock / Broth

Making your own stock is super easy, nourishing and highly versatile. You really just need to throw a few items into a big stockpot and leave it to simmer for several hours. You can even pan roast the bones for a half hour first, which will enhance the flavours and colours but won't change the nutritional value.

Ingredients:

2 kg chicken carcass or wings, or beef/lamb bones
2 carrots, chopped
4 celery stalks, including leaves
1 large onion, chopped
4–6 garlic cloves
2 tbsp apple cider vinegar or juice of 1 lemon
1 tbsp whole black peppercorns
A few sprigs parsley and thyme
2 bay leaves
Salt to taste
2–3 litres water

Instructions:

Place ingredients in a large saucepan, cover with water and bring to boil. Reduce heat and simmer, covered, for 2 hours (up to 24 hours if desired), skimming foam periodically. Strain and chill; remove fat once solidified.

Variations:

1. Freeze in ice-cube trays for small portions.
2. Use as stock cubes for recipes.

Chicken Congee

We love suggesting congee (or chicken and rice porridge) because of its high nutritional value and is just really delicious. Give congee a go especially during the colder months!

Ingredients:

200 g chicken on the bone
1 cup rice
2–4 tsp finely chopped ginger
1 medium onion
4 garlic cloves
Water to cover
2 tsp oil
Salt to taste

Instructions:

Heat oil, cook ginger, garlic, and onion until soft. Add chicken with bone. Cover with water and boil for 15 minutes. Add rice and extra water for porridge consistency. Season with salt. Serve with optional spring onions, sesame oil, parsley, or coriander.

Notes:

- Adjust ginger for children or adults.

Onion Soup – aka French Onion Soup

This is an age-old recipe that is surprisingly filling and provides the whole family with an immune boost. Robyn says her children absolutely love Onion Soup. It is one of the most warming and nourishing winter soups that everyone loves. Be prepared for them to come back for seconds and third helpings. Robyn always doubles or triples this recipe when making it in the eternal hope of having some left over! When sick, this soup is very soothing and nourishing. The onion is beautifully cleansing and helps clear the respiratory tract, release toxins and lower fevers.

Ingredients:

450 g onions, finely sliced
1 litre beef stock
2 garlic cloves, finely minced
½ tsp grated ginger
½ tsp lemon zest
50 g butter
1 tbsp oil
2 tsp honey or sugar
Salt and pepper to taste
1 tbsp plain flour
75 g cheese (Gruyere, goat, or wany cheese of choice)
4 slices toasted bread

Instructions:

Heat oil and butter, add onions, cover and cook gently for 20 minutes, stirring halfway. Add garlic, ginger, lemon zest, flour, and honey. Cook a few minutes to caramelise. Add stock, salt and pepper. Simmer 40 minutes. Grill cheese on toast and serve on top.

Variations:

1. Without cheese croutons, or with softened bread instead.
2. Adult version: add ¾ cup white wine 30 minutes before end, 30 ml brandy 5 minutes before serving.

Miso & Vermicelli Soup

This is one of the easiest and quickest soups to make. Quick, nourishing and easy for lunch or dinner. The whole thing can be done in as little as 10 minutes.

Ingredients (per person):

½ tbsp miso paste
½ bunch rice vermicelli
Small handful leafy greens (baby bok-choy, spinach, or Chinese greens)
1–2 mushrooms
1 cup boiling water

Instructions:

Place ingredients in saucepan, pour boiling water over, and cook 5 minutes until vermicelli soft and vegetables wilted. Add greens last 2 minutes if desired.

Notes:

- Instant miso soup packets can also work e.g. Hikari Miso Instant Miso Soup or Marukome Instant Miso Soup Sachets

Miso & Tofu Soup

Nourishing soup with immune-boosting mushrooms.

Ingredients:

500 ml chicken stock
2 tbsp miso paste
1 carrot, finely julienned
1 bunch bok-choy
2 garlic cloves, finely sliced
1 tsp grated fresh ginger
2 tbsp chopped spring onion greens
1 cayenne pepper (optional)
Soy sauce to taste
100 g silken tofu
1–2 tbsp Immune Mushie Mix*, soaked 20 minutes

*Immune Mushie Mix: combination of dried shiitake, reishi, maitake, turkey tail mushrooms

Instructions:

Bring stock, garlic, and ginger to boil. Add carrot and bok-choy, simmer 2 minutes. Stir in miso paste, soy sauce, and tofu. Stand briefly before serving.

Chickpea & Sweet Potato Soup

Orange vegetables like carrot, sweet potato and pumpkin are high in vitamin A and D and help fight inflammation.

Ingredients:

400 g canned chickpeas
1 sweet potato, chopped
1 cup rice
1 onion, chopped
2–3 slices fresh ginger
2 garlic cloves, chopped and rested 15 minutes
1–2 large tomatoes
½ tsp ground cumin
½ tsp ground cardamom
½ tsp ground coriander
½ tsp fennel seeds
1 chilli (optional)
1 litre water or stock
Fresh parsley and coriander, finely chopped for serving

Instructions:

Fry onion and garlic until soft. Add rice and spices, stir a few minutes. Add chickpeas, sweet potato, tomatoes, and stock. Boil then simmer 20 minutes. Serve with fresh herbs.

Lentil Soup

Hearty, nutrient-rich soup.

Ingredients:

350 g red lentils
2 onions, chopped
2 garlic cloves, chopped
2 carrots, chopped
½ red capsicum, chopped
2 celery sticks, chopped
2 tsp ground cumin
½ tsp ground turmeric
1 tsp ground coriander
2 litres stock
Salt and pepper to taste
2 tbsp olive oil
1 cup spinach, chopped (add last 5 minutes)

Instructions:

Heat oil, fry onions and garlic until soft. Add spices 1–2 minutes. Add remaining ingredients, bring to boil, then simmer 30 minutes. Add spinach last 5 minutes.

Vichyssoise – Potato and Leek Soup (Pumpkin Variation Optional)

Smooth, creamy, and versatile.

Ingredients:

2 leeks, sliced
1 large onion, peeled and diced
750 g potatoes (or 500 g potatoes + 750g pumpkin if making the pumpkin variation)
1 litre chicken stock
1 tbsp butter or oil
1¼ cups cream or Greek yoghurt
Salt and pepper to taste
Parsley, chives, or spring onion for garnish

Instructions:

Sweat leeks and onions in butter or oil until soft. Add potatoes (and pumpkin), cover with stock, boil, then simmer 25 minutes. Blend smooth. Add cream and simmer 5 minutes. Add yoghurt after cooking if using. Garnish.

Variations:

Pumpkin, sweet potato or bacon variations

Green Soup

Nourishing, green vegetable soup with immune support.

Ingredients:

1 onion
2 garlic cloves
small piece ginger, finely chopped
1 zucchini
2 celery stalks, chopped
½ bunch flat-leaf parsley
including stalks
100 g baby spinach leaves
½ cup frozen green peas or beans
1 bunch broccolini, chopped
2 medium potatoes
6 dried shiitake mushrooms, pre-soaked 20 minutes
1 tbsp cashew butter
1 tbsp beef broth
1 litre beef or vegetable stock
400 g canned white cannellini beans, drained and rinsed
2 tbsp oil
Salt and pepper to taste

Instructions:

Chop all vegetables into small pieces. Heat oil, cook onion and ginger until soft. Add potato, mushrooms, garlic, and celery for 5 minutes. Add remaining ingredients except spinach, boil, simmer 20–25 minutes. Add spinach and cook until wilted. Blend until smooth.

Notes:

- Can add cream or dairy substitute

Substitute:

Blend together equal quantities of Silken Tofu and Soy milk. This can be used for soups, quiches, and can be whipped for cakes etc.

Carrot, Capsicum, and Ginger Soup

This is not only a delicious soup, but it is very nourishing and immune boosting. Kids will generally enjoy it as the carrots make it quite sweet.

Ingredients:

2 cups chicken broth
500 g carrots, peeled and chopped
1 tsp grated ginger
1 small red onion
1 garlic clove
1 tbsp oil
1 cup water
Pinch fresh thyme leaves

Instructions:

Heat oil, cook onion, garlic and ginger until soft. Add carrots, stock, water, and thyme. Simmer 30–40 minutes. Blend smooth.

Chickpea & Avocado Dip

Nutritious and creamy dip.

Ingredients:

200 g chickpeas
2 ripe avocados, peeled and pitted
2 tbsp tahini
3 tbsp olive oil
1 garlic clove
3 tbsp lemon juice
½ tsp cumin
Small amount chilli flakes or fresh chopped chilli (optional)
Salt and pepper to taste
Fresh parsley to sprinkle

Instructions:

Blend chickpeas, tahini, olive oil, garlic, lemon juice and cumin until smooth. Add avocado and pulse until well blended. Season and serve with parsley.

Guacamole

Avocados are packed full of healthy oils and vitamins. Guacamole can be used as a dip with fresh carrot and celery sticks. Even when your child is sick, you can be guaranteed that they are getting a nutritious snack. Use it as a topping to a meal like tacos or burritos, with potato skins (see recipe below) or an addition to salads.

Ingredients:

1 ripe avocado, mashed
Juice of 1 lemon
2–3 sprigs chopped parsley
2–3 sprigs chopped chives or spring onion
1–2 garlic cloves, crushed
1 small tomato, finely chopped (optional)
2–4 tbsp yoghurt or sour cream

Instructions:

Mash avocado with lemon juice. Add remaining ingredients. Serve with raw vegetables or as a meal topping.

Potato Skins

Potatoes hold a lot of their nutrients just under the skin. This recipe takes advantage of these nutrients. Skin your potatoes about 1cm thick. Use the remaining potato in soups or as mash, or cut into small wedges.

Ingredients:

Potato skins cut 1 cm thick
Bacon, diced and fried
Sour cream
Guacamole
Grated cheese
Chopped parsley

Instructions:

Bake potato skins at 220°C for ~30 minutes until golden. Layer with bacon and cheese, bake 5 minutes more. Top with guacamole, sour cream, and parsley.

Hummus with Carrot Sticks

Classic chickpea dip.

Ingredients:

1 can chickpeas, drained (keep some liquid in case you need it when blending)
1 garlic clove
¼ cup tahini paste
Juice of ½ lemon
Carrot sticks

Instructions:

Blend all ingredients until smooth. Add chickpea liquid as needed. Serve with olive oil drizzle and paprika.

Gooey Celery Sticks and Apple Chunks

Peanut butter, almond butter and other nut spreads make celery sticks and apple slices fun to eat.

Ingredients:

Celery sticks
Apples, cored and sliced
Peanut, almond, or cashew butter
Cream cheese (optional)

Instructions:

Spread nut butter or cream cheese into celery groove or on apple slices.

Notes:

- A slinky machine cuts apples and other hard fruits or vegetables into coils. It becomes a novelty and kids will often eat the foods they 'slinky' that they might otherwise refuse.

Chippies

What kid won't eat chippies even when they are sick? These delicious hot chips are not only easy to make but they are also guilt free especially to give to the little ones as they are baked in the oven or air fryer, and are not full of fat.

Ingredients:

1 sweet potato
2 potatoes
1 parsnip
¼ small pumpkin
1 medium beetroot
3 garlic cloves, whole with skin
Oil for brushing
Salt and rosemary (optional)

Instructions:

Preheat oven 250°C. Cut vegetables into chip sizes. Lightly coat with oil, bake until golden, turning once. Add salt/rosemary or as desired.

Notes:

- Sage is also another good herb to use, roughly chopped. This herb is antibacterial and can help fight any infections causing fevers.

Healthy Mash

Nutritious vegetable mash which are perfect accompaniments to many dishes.

Ingredients:

1 potato
1 sweet potato
2 carrots
Pumpkin, fist size
1 cup chicken or beef stock
1 clove garlic, optional
Butter for mashing
Parsley, finely chopped
Spring onion, optional

Instructions:

Cook vegetables in stock until soft. Blend, add butter, garnish with parsley and spring onion (or sour cream or yoghurt when serving). Optional: add garlic last minute.

Baked Beans

This classic staple is in fact considered a super food. Baked beans are full of protein, fibre and iron, which are good for protecting against heart disease and many cancers. Of course, many other beans and pulses fall into this category too and can be easily swapped for the usual cannelloni beans in this recipe.

Ingredients:

400 g canned cannelloni beans, washed and drained
250 g tomatoes, fresh or canned
2 tbsp olive oil
1 small purple onion, chopped
1 garlic clove, chopped
1 cup water
1 tsp paprika
½ tsp cumin
2 tbsp chopped parsley
1 tbsp coconut sugar
Salt to taste

Instructions:

Cook onion and garlic in olive oil until soft. Add remaining ingredients and cook 20 minutes on low heat. Serve with hot buttered toast.

Osso Bucco

A great one-pot meal you can put on in the morning and let slowly cook, ready for dinner at night. Because it has been slow-cooked, the meat is easier to digest and the marrow from the bones infuses this dish with nourishing goodness. Top it with some gremolata for a nutritious parsley and lemon vitamin-filled, flavourful garnish.

Ingredients:

1 kg osso bucco pieces
2 medium-sized red onions, chopped
2 cloves garlic, minced
2 large carrots, roughly chopped
2 sticks celery, finely chopped
1 small sweet potato
50 g tomato paste
1 can tomato pieces
500 ml beef stock
2 tablespoons olive oil
Plain flour, to toss osso bucco in
1 tablespoon plain flour
2 bay leaves
6 peppercorns

Gremolata:

Fresh parsley
Lemon zest

Instructions:

Toss the osso bucco pieces in plain flour and shake off the excess. In a saucepan, add 1 tablespoon of oil and brown the osso bucco pieces. Remove and set aside. Add the remaining oil to the pan, then add the onions and garlic. Cook until the onions are soft. Add the tomatoes, tomato paste, beef stock, and osso bucco pieces. Bring to the boil. Cover and simmer for 1½ to 2 hours. Add the vegetables, season with salt, and simmer for another 20–30 minutes, until the vegetables are soft. Serve and sprinkle with gremolata.

Tuna Casserole

A classic, hearty, family-friendly casserole that's simple to prepare and full of comforting flavour.

Ingredients:

425 g tin tuna in brine or spring water – retain liquid for sauce
1 medium-large onion, diced and sautéed in butter
1 cup peas
1 carrot, diced

Sauce:
60 g butter
3 tablespoons flour
2 cups milk
175 g grated cheese
pinch of pepper

Topping:
3 slices of bread, cut into cubes
Butter, melted
Extra cheese

Instructions:

Drain the liquid from the tuna and reserve it for the sauce. Place the vegetables and tuna in a deep casserole dish. Melt the butter in a large saucepan and add the flour. Cook for a few minutes, then remove from heat. Gradually stir in the milk and the reserved tuna liquid. Return to heat and slowly bring to a boil, stirring all the time to avoid burning. Add the grated cheese and pepper, stirring until the sauce is smooth. Pour the sauce over the tuna and vegetables.

Melt butter in a saucepan, add the cubed bread and stir until all pieces are lightly coated. Place the buttered bread cubes on top of the tuna mixture and sprinkle with extra cheese. Cook in a moderate oven (180°C) for 20–30 minutes.

Tuna, Spaghetti and Mushroom Mornay

Robyn says: "This is a quick and easy standby, which my kids and their friends always like, even when they aren't eating other foods as readily. It doesn't take long to prepare or cook. My kids will happily have this cold in their lunch boxes. It was one of the first meals they learned to prepare for themselves."

Ingredients:

1 tin cream of mushroom soup (Campbell's brand works best)
1 grated onion (chopped is too strong-flavoured)
¾ cup milk
425 g tin tuna, drained
2 cups cooked macaroni or spirals
½ cup buttered bread cubes (see note)
1 tablespoon grated cheese (more if you like)

Instructions:

In a large, shallow greased casserole dish, mix the soup, grated onion and milk. Add the flaked tuna and cooked macaroni. Sprinkle the top with buttered bread cubes and cheese. Bake uncovered in a moderate oven (180°C or 375°F) for 20–30 minutes.

Note on Buttered Bread Cubes:

Dice or cube 2–3 slices of bread (a good way to use crust ends). Place the bread cubes in a small amount of butter in a saucepan and toss until lightly coated but not saturated.

Optional Extra:

Add ½ to 1 cup frozen peas when you add the tuna.

FOOD FOR THOUGHT

In the journey of healing, food is more than just sustenance, it is medicine. If you have none of the listed remedies in this book, you can still support your child's healing with the recipes. The recipes gathered here are designed to help heal and nourish the body, to support the immune system, and to aid in the healing process during any illness and recovery period. It's not just about healing the physical body but also about nurturing the mind and spirit.

By embracing the healing power of food, you are taking an active role in your child's health, using every meal as an opportunity to support their body's natural ability to heal and regenerate. The beauty of these recipes lies in their adaptability, they are meant to serve as a guide, allowing you to create meals that are healing and delicious.

Using these recipes when your child is sick, not only will you feel empowered, but you are also teaching your children that there are things that they can do to feel better and recover more quickly when they are ill. Robyn has used some of these recipes since her children were little and as young children they would often request them. Even now as young adults she often sees them making these recipes for themselves when they are not feeling well.

When you include some of these recipes in your meal plan, you can help establish long-term healthy eating habits. While designed with healing and recovery in mind, many of the principles focus on whole, unprocessed foods, minimising inflammatory ingredients, and incorporating a variety of nutrient-dense plants which are beneficial for overall health and wellbeing. By continuing to eat in this health-focused way even after your child has recovered, you can maintain the strength and resilience in their body, supporting their immune system and potentially preventing future illness.

Ultimately, the recipes in this collection are more than just food, they are a form of self-care, a way to support the body through its healing process. By nourishing your child and family with these healing foods, you are laying the groundwork for a healthy, vibrant future.

Afterword

In *Treating Fever Without Fear: Natural Remedies for Health and Wellbeing*, we have shared many time-tested approaches with you including many natural remedies that can help you to safely, effectively and successfully manage fevers without feeling fearful. From Herbal Remedies, Tissue Salts, Homeopathic Remedies and Healthy Food Recipes, you will be equipped with tools to navigate fever episodes for you and your children confidently.

Throughout this book, we've explored the nature of fever, delved into the body's remarkable self-healing capabilities, and discovered the power of natural remedies.

One of the themes of our book is to remind you that Fever is not an enemy to be feared, it is a natural and essential part of the healing process. By understanding this, you can shift your mindset from anxiety and fear to trust and confidence. Remember, the body knows how to heal itself, and fever is a process not an illness, and is in fact, an essential tool in helping the body fight illness.

In this light, our role as parents and caregivers always changes. Instead of rushing to suppress fever at the first sign of a raised temperature, we can take a more measured and informed approach. We can observe, support, and provide comfort, trusting that the body is doing what it needs to do to fight off illness and restore balance.

You understand when it's appropriate to let the fever run its course, when to use natural remedies for relief, and when to seek medical attention if necessary. This balanced approach empowers you to make the best decisions for your child's health, based on both modern medical knowledge and time-honoured natural practices.

Throughout our book, we have explored various natural remedies that can be used to support the body during a fever. These remedies work in harmony with the body's natural processes rather than against them, in conjunction with proper hydration, and nourishing foods. The remedies we share with you will not only help to alleviate discomfort but also help strengthen the immune system, promoting long-term health and resilience.

This book is more than just a guide to managing fever, it's a call to action to change the way you think about illness and health. By embracing the concepts in our book, you can move away from fear-based reactions and toward a more holistic, nurturing approach to caregiving.

Imagine a future where parents everywhere feel equipped and confident in caring for their children during a fever. A future where natural remedies are widely recognised and used as a first line of support and healing, and where the body's natural healing processes are respected. This is the vision we hope to inspire.

As you close this book, remember that the journey doesn't end here. The knowledge you've gained is just the beginning. Remember that you can pull our book off of your shelf and use it whenever your child has fever. Write on it and make notes and observations until it becomes dog eared and worn! Share copies with your friends and continue to educate yourself about natural health practices, stay connected with healthcare professionals who respect your approach, and share what you've learned with others.

Most importantly, trust yourself. You are your child's best advocate and caregiver. With the tools and understanding you've gained from *Treating Fever Without Fear*, you can approach fever and illness with confidence, compassion and a deep sense of empowerment.

Thank you for taking this journey with us. Together, we can create a world where fever is no longer feared but understood and embraced as a natural part of the healing process. Here's to a future of fearless, informed and holistic caregiving.

About the Authors

Molly Knight

Dip. Nutr., Dip. Irid., Dip. CHt., Grad. Dip Herbal Med.

Molly is a true pioneer in the field of Healing. After leaving school Molly trained as a nurse before becoming ill herself, and after a long search, she was healed using natural remedies. Her healing journey sparked a profound shift in her life's purpose, which incited her to change her path and qualify in natural methods of healing.

As a renowned clinical practitioner with over 43 years in the natural health field, Molly has worked with thousands of individuals helping them tap into their own innate healing abilities. The tenure as a lecturer at Nature Care College in Sydney further amplified her influence as she educated and empowered students with a vast knowledge, unique blend of healing modalities and practical techniques.

Molly's expertise encompasses a wide range of disciplines including Herbal Medicine, Homeopathy, and Nutrition, as well as Clinical Hypnotherapy, Meditation, Qi Gong and Emotional Freedom Technique (EFT). This rich and diverse toolkit has allowed Molly to facilitate profound shifts in the lives of those she has touched, guiding them towards greater health and wellbeing.

Molly's passion for healing extended beyond her one-on-one work with patients. She is also an accomplished educator offering courses that cover a broad spectrum of topics related to health and wellness. The courses include Emotional Healing, Body Cleansing and Healing, Pathway To Healing (Cancer Support), Winter Health for Children, Meditation and Visualisation, EFT, Energy Healing and Create Your Day. These courses have empowered countless individuals to take control of their health and wellbeing, providing them with the tools and knowledge to heal themselves.

Although Molly has retired from clinical practice, her dedication to healing remains as strong as ever, as she continues to work online, supporting cancer and chronically ill patients, helping their body and mind strengthen after they have completed their medical treatments. Molly periodically runs a Healing Circle support group for individual suffering from cancer and chronic illness, offering a space for connection, healing, and hope, providing ongoing support and inspiration to those who need it most. Having personally experienced cancer, Molly dedicates herself to guiding and supporting others on their road to recovery.

Molly is also a prolific author having written several books that reflect her deep knowledge and passion for natural health. The publications include the Create Your Day series (Books 1, 2 and 3), Allergy Link to Illness, Allergy Free Sweet Treats, Pathway to Healing, along with her love of writing children's books, Dr. Gott Gott, a children's picture book series, and three colouring in books, Happy Critters Affirmations and Gratitude Kids Colouring and Drawing Book, and two Christmas themed Colouring and Activity Books.

Through her writing, Molly continues to share her wisdom and insights, reaching a global audience and helping people of all ages on their journeys to health and wellbeing. Molly's legacy is one of compassion, wisdom and a relentless commitment to the healing of others. Her work continues to inspire and transform, leaving a lasting impact on all who encounter her teachings.

Molly can be found on her YouTube Channel called 'The Healing Path'.

Robyn Barraclough (Pfitzner)

BA Comm, Adv. Dip. Classical Herbal Med (Dorothy Hall), Dip. Natural Medicines, Dip. Clinical Science of Biochemic Medicine

Robyn Barraclough is a Herbalist, Homeopath, Body Harmony Practitioner, and educator who has spent over 25 years helping families navigate health challenges with confidence instead of fear. As a Teacher of Tissue Salts for over 15 years and Body Harmony for over 20 years, she has also presented at National and International Conferences, including Practitioner training for 'The Clinical Science of Biochemic Medicine', and Tissue Salts Diploma Course in conjunction with the Institute of Biochemic Medicine (Asia-Pacific) and online at www.tissuesaltstraining.com.

Her work bridges the connection between body chemistry and body awareness—helping people understand how physical symptoms are linked to emotional states. Through Tissue Salts, she provides the body with essential minerals for healing, while her somatic-based Body Harmony practice supports the release of stored tension, trauma, and fear that can keep people stuck in cycles of illness or anxiety.

She brings a sense of humour and realness to her workshops, making complex concepts accessible, practical, and deeply transformative for her clients and students.

Robyn's path into natural medicine emerged from growing herbs as a teenager and learning all she could about using them medicinally and in cooking. The birth of her first daughter inspired her career change, going deeper into Herbal Medicine, Homeopathy and Body Harmony, a form of body mind hands-on bodywork, and was hooked. Robyn has maintained a practice since 2000, alongside the real-world learning and beautiful chaos of raising five children, including twins.

Her approach has always been deeply practical. She understands that parents need clear answers in the middle of the night, not philosophy. They need to know: What remedy? What dose? When do I worry? When do I wait? This book is born from thousands of those moments—both in her own home and in her clinical practice.

When her one of her 16-year-old twin daughters was diagnosed with a high-grade, fast-growing inoperable brain cancer, Robyn faced the reality of when to trust natural remedies, when medical intervention was necessary, and how to integrate both for the best possible outcome. This experience deepened her understanding of how fear affects the body—and how to move beyond it. She learned to navigate the complex terrain between natural remedies and medical intervention, understanding that true healing wisdom isn't about choosing one over the other, but knowing when each is called for.

Her daughter Alana has defied the odds and is in the less than 5% of children/adults still alive after her diagnosis. Despite the tumour recurring in 2024, at the end of 2025 it's stable and even shrinking slightly. Whilst she still has effects, she is living a life, close to normal, currently without need for medication, and is completely astounding the medical fraternity.

Fever is a large concern in many cancer patients. She used the protocols in this book, in consultation with specialists, especially the Tissue Salts and Homoeopathics to reduce severity and length of fever, when it didn't conflict with access to chosen medical treatment.

What makes Robyn's work unique is her integration of physical biochemistry with somatic (body-based) therapy. Through her training in Body Harmony—a modality that recognizes how the body holds tension, trauma, and emotional patterns in its very tissues—she helps people release stuck emotions, to live lives more aligned with their inner truth and desires.

A child's recurring fever might be the body's inflammatory response to a virus, yes—but it might also be amplified by stored stress in the nervous system, by unprocessed fear, by the anxiety they're picking up from a worried parent. This is why Robyn teaches parents not just what remedy to give, but how to regulate their own nervous system first. When you're calm, your child feels safer. When your child feels safer, their body can focus on healing instead of defending against perceived threat. It's beautifully simple, though not always easy to do, and it changes everything.

Today, when she teaches parents how to treat fever naturally, she does so with the hard-won wisdom of someone who has stood in the gap between natural remedies and appropriate medical intervention. She believes that fever is not something to be feared but a sign of the body's intelligence at work, and she teaches families and practitioners how to support the body's natural processes rather than suppress them.

Outside of her work, Robyn loves writing, music and dancing and has embraced creativity through burlesque performance, scriptwriting, and film production as part of The Writers Formerly Known As....

You can learn more about Robyn and Molly's work here:

Tissue Salts Training

Robyn has taught the Tissue Salts Diploma Course in conjunction with the Institute of Biochemic Medicine (Asia-Pacific), both online and in workshops, training practitioners in 'The Clinical Science of Biochemic Medicine'. Her students include naturopaths, herbalists, kinesiologists, nurses, midwives, and parents who wanted deeper knowledge to care for their families.

What her students consistently report is that Robyn makes complex biochemistry accessible and practical. She doesn't just teach which Tissue Salt does what, she teaches facial diagnosis, so you can see mineral deficiencies written on the face. She teaches the "why" behind the protocols, so you're not just following recipes but truly understanding how the body works at a cellular level.

Her teaching style blends rigorous science with storytelling, clinical precision with warmth and humour. As one student put it: "Robyn has a treasure chest of knowledge and a great sense of humour too. The most enjoyable course as well as a must for all Natural therapy professionals."

Find out more about Tissue Salts Practitioner Training at https://tissuesaltstraining.com/

Robyn also has online courses to help you treat your family naturally with Tissue Salts at https://tissuesaltstraining.com/tissue-salts-for-everyday-enroll/

Suburban Goddess – Women's Empowerment

Robyn's journey through her daughter's cancer diagnosis and her divorce led her to a powerful realization: we spend so much of our lives following the "good girl" script, doing what we're supposed to, caring for everyone else, pushing down our own desires and dreams, that we forget how to truly live.

This awakening sparked another dimension of her work: Suburban Goddess, a transformational space for women who are ready to ditch the 'good girl' conditioning, reclaim their power, and create lives that genuinely light them up. It's about permission to take up space, to prioritize joy, to stop shrinking themselves to make others comfortable. https://suburban-goddess.com/

Wise Women's Wellness – The Natural Medicine Cabinet

Robyn and Molly are 2 Wise Women with a wealth of wellness knowledge to share, to help you create your natural medicine cabinet, and to teach you how to use those remedies for a variety of ailments. Look out for more books and courses on a broad range of topics. Stay posted at https://bodyharmony.com.au/ .

Find out more about Treating Fever at https://bodyharmony.com.au/www-treatingfever/

References and Resources

Fever

1. 'Fever Management, evidence vs current practice' https://www.ncbi.nlm.nih.gov/pmc/articles/

PMC4145646/, A.Sahib Mehdi El-Radhi, World Journal of Clinical Paediatrics, accessed 10/08/23

2. 'Fever: suppress it or let it ride?' Juliet J Ray and Carl I.Schulman, https://www.ncbi.nlm.nih.gov/pmc/articles/PMC4703655/, Journal of Thoracic Disease, 2015, Dec, 7

3. 'Fever Management, Evidence vs Current Practice' World Journal of Clinical Paediatrics El-Radhi.

Dr MD, Vikas Sharma MD, 7 Best Homeopathic medicines for Fever

Tissue Salts

Peter Emmrich 'Facial Diagnostics, An introduction to the Biochemic Healing Method of Dr Schuessler, Weg zur Gesundheit Verlag GmbH, Dormagen, Germany

Gunther H.Heepen, Schuessler Tissue Salts, 12 Minerals for Your Health", Deutsche Homeopathie Union

The Institute of Biochemic Medicine (Asia Pacific) , 'The Clinical Science of Biochemic Therapy Diploma Course'

The Institute of Biochemic Medicine (Asia Pacific), 'Advanced Biochemistry of Dr W. H. Schuessler, the Supplementary Biochemic Remedies'

Herbal Medicine

Matthew Wood, 'The Book of Herbal Wisdom' North Atlanta Books, Berkeley California, 1997

Matthew Wood with David Ryan, 'The Earthwise Herbal Repertory, the Definitive Practitioner's Guide', North Atlantic Books Berkeley California, 2016

Matthew Wood, 'The Earthwise Herbal, A Complete Guide to Old World Medicinal Plants", North Atlantic Books, Berkeley, California, 2008

Dorothy Hall, 'Dorothy Hall's Herbal Medicine', A Lothian Book, Port Melbourne, Victoria, 1995

Prasanta Banerji, Pratip Banaji, 'the Banaji Protocols, A new method of Treatment with Homeopathic Medicines', Dr Prasanta Banerji Research Foundation, West Bengal, India, 2013